# THE HEALING OF CANCER

## The Cures, the Cover-ups and the Solution Now

**BY BARRY LYNES**

First printing May 1989
Second printing December 1990
Third printing August 1995

* * *

Published in Canada by Marcus books,
P.O.Box 327, Queensville, Ontario,
Canada L0G 1R0. (905) 478-2201
Fax: (905) 478-8338

ISBN 0-919951-44-9

* * *

Cover design by W. G. Meakins

Printed in Canada by Webcom Ltd.

## Disclaimer

This book is not intended to replace the services of a physician. It is a critical examination of orthodox, alternative and potential cancer therapies as well as a look at the politics of cancer. Any use of the information set forth in the following pages is at the reader's discretion. No statement included in this book should be taken as medical advice. The author and publisher assume no responsibility for any decision made by the reader regarding cancer treatment.

Barry Lynes has authored three books on the subject of Cancer:

The Cancer Cure that Worked
The Healing of Cancer
Helping the Cancer Victim

These books are available from the publisher:
Marcus Books, P.O. Box 327, Queensville,
Ontario, Canada L0G 1R0
Tel: (416) 478-2201; FAX (416) 478-8338

"I swear by Apollo the physician . . . I will keep this Oath
. . .

"I will follow that system of regimen which, according to
my ability and judgment, I consider for the benefit of my
patients, and abstain from whatever is deleterious and mis-
chievous.

"I will give no deadly medicine to anyone . . .

"Into whatever houses I enter, I will go into them for the
benefit of the sick, and will abstain from every voluntary act
of mischief and corruption . . ."

The Oath of Hippocrates, the Father
of Medicine

"Cancer deaths and incidents in the United States are at an
all-time high . . . . Yet there is evidence that all the potential
help that alternative therapies could offer has been and is still
being suppressed."

*The Guardian* of London, September 29, 1990,
One of England's leading newspapers.

# CONTENTS

# Introduction

Dr. James Watson won a Nobel Prize for determining the shape of DNA. During the 1970s, he served two years on the National Cancer Advisory Board. In 1975, he was asked about the National Cancer Program. He declared, "It's a bunch of shit."[1]

In 1953, a United States Senate Investigation reported that a conspiracy existed to suppress effective cancer treatments. The Senator in charge of the investigation conveniently died. The investigation was halted. It was neither the first nor the last of a number of strange deaths involving people in positions to do damage to those running the nation's cancer program.[2]

In 1964, the Food and Drug Administration (FDA) spent millions of dollars to stop an alternative cancer treatment which had cured hundreds, if not thousands, of cancer patients according to documented records. It was later disclosed that FDA had falsified the testimony of witnesses. FDA lost the court case because the jury found the defendants innocent and recommended that the substance be objectively evaluated. It never was. Instead, it was totally suppressed.[3]

In the early 1960s, two New York City doctors, one associated with the leading cancer center in America and the other the medical director of a Brooklyn hospital, decided to inject live cancer cells into 22 unknowing patients. When they were discovered, Dr. Chester M. Southam of the Memorial Sloan-Kettering Cancer Center and Dr. E. E. Mandel of the Jewish Chronic Disease Hospital of Brooklyn were put on "probation" for a year. The three physicians who "blew the whistle" on Dr. Southam and Dr. Mandel were dismissed.[4]

For many years, the American Medical Association (AMA)

1

and the American Cancer Society (ACS) coordinated their "hit" lists of innovative cancer researchers who were to be ostracized. One investigative reporter declared the AMA and ACS "form a network of vigilantes prepared to pounce on anyone who promotes a cancer therapy that runs against their substantial prejudices and profits."[5]

In the late 1950s, it was learned that Dr. Henry Welch, head of the FDA's Division of Antibiotics, had secretly received $287,000 from the drug companies he was supposed to regulate. In 1975, an independent government evaluation of FDA still found massive "conflicts of interest" among the agency's top personnel.[6]

In 1977, an investigative team from the prominent Long Island newspaper *Newsday* found serious "conflicts of interest" at the National Cancer Institute (NCI). In 1986, an organized cover-up of an effective alternative cancer therapy, orchestrated by NCI officials, was revealed during Congressional hearings.

These examples are only the tip of a huge iceberg. The cancer establishment now has a 50-year history of vast corruption, incompetence and organized suppression of cancer therapies which actually work. Millions of people have suffered terrible torture and death because those in charge took payoffs, played it safe, had closed minds to the innovative, or simply were afraid to do what was obviously and morally right.

This book will shock many, especially those who have cancer and are seeking a cure. The total healing of cancer is possible. I do not mislead you on that. The title of this book is accurate. The methods are described in this book. But it is important to emphasize *again and again and again* that finding a cure is not the problem. The cures for many cancers, if not most cancers, exist. But they are not being offered to the patient who has cancer.

It must be emphasized, however, that a cancer therapy which works on one type of cancer may not be effective with another. Some careful evaluation needs to be done in determining which alternative, *suppressed* cancer treatments work for which types of cancer. But again, finding a cure is not the

2

problem. *Being legally permitted to use an alternative cancer therapy is the problem.* This is where the struggle lies. And any concerned citizen or cancer patient who is not aware of that simple fact will miss the message and the *call to action* of this book.

The doctor's union (AMA), the cancer bureaucracy (NCI), the public relations fatcats (ACS) and the cancer cops (FDA) are conspiring to suppress a cure for cancer. That is an accusation which is not made lightly and it is certainly one that the reader will not accept without evidence. This book presents numerous examples and explanations of how the conspiracy operates. It would be easy for any Congressional committee, major newspaper, television network or national magazine to confirm and extend the evidence presented here in order to initiate radical reform of the critical cancer arenas—the hospitals, the research centers, the government agencies, and especially state and local legislation regarding cancer treatment.

But that will not happen without a struggle. Neither Congress nor the media desire to lift the manhole cover on this sewer of corruption and needless torture. Only organized, determined citizen opposition to the existing cancer treatment system has any hope of bringing about the long-needed changes. I expect the struggle to be a long, difficult one against tough, murderous opposition. The odds against success are heavy. The vested interests are very powerful.

I have accused here some of the most powerful institutions in America and some of the most powerful people in America of a conscious conspiracy to suppress cancer therapies which work. Naturally they will ignore my indictment or, if forced, will respond with self-serving defenses regarding their past behavior, be it personal or institutional. In time, as the truth of what I have described here in late 1988 becomes accepted knowledge, then those who perpetrated the crimes will offer more elaborate excuses. Ignorance should be prominent among their alibis. I warn my future readers not to be brainwashed.

Thousands of doctors, radiologists, nurses, researchers, bureaucrats, members of Congress, their Congressional assistants and numerous journalists have known what has been

3

going on for years. Millions of people have been mutilated, tortured and murdered while those who could have spoken out remained silent. Obviously a few did speak. A Nobel Prize winner such as Dr. James Watson could use the most vulgar putdown to characterize the entire National Cancer Program, "It's a bunch of shit," and yet no high level media or governmental attempt to change the situation resulted. Other scientists and independent journalists could "blow the whistle" on various aspects of the cancer conspiracy, yet again no change resulted, no matter how outrageous the crime exposed or the number of people killed because of it. The fix was in. It has existed for a long time and woe to those who challenged it.

I believe the reason why this murderous state of affairs exists is simple. It has two primary parts. The first is that those in charge of the conspiracy are extremely powerful and thus those in a position to challenge them are reluctant to risk their lives or careers in order to do so. Second, I believe we live in conservative, status-quo times characterized by cowardice instead of courage from our political leaders.

This is not a book on mass psychology or the need for heroes and heroines, but it is worth noting that great wrongs usually require courageous acts by courageous men and women if a downward spiral into further debasement and evil is to be prevented. I personally believe that the cancer establishment is fundamentally corrupt and is now threatening the nation's very survival.

Having stated clearly that it is my opinion that a conspiracy exists, it needs to be emphasized that the criticisms in this book are *not* directed at the numerous dedicated doctors and researchers who sincerely seek a cure for cancer. Many of these professionals are so focused on their patients or their particular area of research that they are unaware of the larger political evil and the hidden activities by faceless men and women in the corridors of power—the deals which kill millions of people, the legal language that gives a drug company an exemption from FDA rules, the covert moves against alternative therapies—indictments, beatings, attempted murder and murder—which result in the therapy's total eradication, the

4

clinical trials at the leading medical centers which are rigged, the blacklists, the mysterious deaths of critics, and so forth.

I am certain that many dedicated physicians and researchers will be surprised by what they learn in these pages. It is to be hoped that these facts will stimulate a revolt "in the ranks", and support for systems which encourage honest evaluation of alternative, non-toxic therapies.

In the following pages, I make my case. I thank you for taking the time to consider my argument.

Barry Lynes
Cupertino, California

Chapter One

# Blood and Money

*"There is not one, but many cures for cancer available.
But they are all being systematically suppressed."*
Robert C. Atkins, M.D.[7]

Every half-hour, 30 people die of cancer in America. Every day, 1400 people die of cancer in America. Every week, almost 10,000 people die of cancer in America. Every year, almost 500,000 people die of cancer in America. Approximately 900,000 Americans will learn this year that they have cancer. Of those, only 40% will be alive in 5 years. (Critics of the national cancer program say only 20%-25%.)

According to James E. Easton of UCLA's School of Public Health, if current trends continue, by the year 2000, 41% of Americans will develop cancer within their lifetimes. A more conservative estimate is that, of 240 million Americans now alive, 74 million will get cancer sometime during their lives unless a breakthrough in cancer prevention or cancer treatment appears.

With such a huge proportion of the American public at risk, it would seem that every media outlet and politician would be committed to open discussion of the problem while supporting a broad examination of alternative treatments. But that is not the situation. There is a virtual press blackout on the subject. Congress refuses to investigate, as will be described later. With no focused attention, those who do actively oppose the health officials and profiteers responsible for the crime are isolated and ignored. Meanwhile, another 1400 die today, with another 1400 scheduled for tomorrow, and another 1400 the day after, on and on. The press runs panic stories about AIDS, almost on a daily basis, speculating about a future epidemic

7

while the epidemic that is here now, and has been for decades, is ignored. Why?

The answer is simple. The cancer industry, including treatment and research, is conservatively estimated to be an annual $50 billion to $75 billion industry. It is a powerful monster out of control that government officials and media barons fear to confront. Hospitals blithely install multi-million dollar radiation devices, knowing they will profit from them while ignoring their murderous effects. Surgeons cut and cut and cut, with meager results, but high fees. Chemotherapists promote more expensive and more toxic cancer "cocktails" which have little effect, as detailed research proves. The few voices of protest are lost in the huge, obscene feeding of the cancer industry profiteers.

According to Arizona State University professor Edward J. Sylvester:

> "The physical plant of what is called the University of Texas (UT) System Cancer Center here covers two million square feet. . . . Current investment in the building is $152 million. The operating budget, separate from physical-plant cost, was $254,389,314 ($254 million!) . . . for fiscal 1984-85. . . . All for cancer. The UT System Cancer Center treats no other disease . . .
>
> "A noted cancer specialist in Boston said he believed that if some simple and inexpensive replacement for chemotherapy for the treatment of cancer were found tomorrow, all U.S. medical schools would teeter on the verge of bankruptcy, so integral a part of their hospital revenues is oncology, the medical specialty of cancer treatment."[8]

The average cost per cancer patient is $50,000–$75,000 and rising. Yet many die of the treatment! As is admitted by a few of the more courageous physicians and researchers.

As early as 1956, Hardin Jones, Ph.D., a professor of medical physics and physiology at the University of California, Berkeley, argued that orthodox cancer treatment (radiation, surgery and chemotherapy) was suspect. In 1969, Jones declared that, according to his carefully researched statistics, the cancer patient who received no treatment had a greater life expectancy than the one who received treatment:

8

"For a typical type of cancer, people who refused treatment live an average of twelve and a half years. Those who accepted surgery and other kinds of treatment lived an average of only three years. I attribute this to the traumatic effect of surgery on the body's natural defense mechanism. The body has a natural kind of defense against every type of cancer."[9]

In 1977, Jones testified in a San Diego hearing that a woman with breast cancer who had *no treatment* lived up to *four times* longer than one who was treated by conventional methods.[10]

Yet the cancer authorities ignored such conclusions by an eminent researcher. The American Cancer Society (ACS), in this author's opinion essentially a corrupt public relations scam, which spends two-thirds of its money on non-research salaries and expenses, continued to promote X-ray examinations for women and traditional treatment for breast cancer.

The conclusions of Berkeley's Hardin Jones deserve widespread dissemination and modern, updated analysis, particularly in light of the link between the American Cancer Society's fund-raising operation for its own institutional interests and its promotion of the idea that early detection of breast cancer leads to extension of life. Jones wrote in 1969:

"In the matter of duration of malignant tumors before treatment, no studies have established the much talked about relationship between early detection and favorable survival after treatment. . . . The possibility exists that treatment makes the average situation worse."[9]

In 1975, the respected British medical journal *Lancet* reported on a study which compared the effect on cancer patients of (1) a single chemotherapy, (2) multiple chemotherapy, and (3) *no treatment at all*. No treatment "proved a significantly better policy for patients' survival and for quality of remaining life."

Then in 1988 a Swedish study found that mammograms (X-rays of breasts) and early detection of breast cancer did not reduce death. Dr. Lars Janzon of Sweden's Malmo General Hospital studied 42,000 women before concluding in an October 1988 *British Medical Journal* that mammograms should be restricted. An official of the American Cancer Society immediately dismissed the report when asked about it by the *Wall Street Journal*.

Not only have health officials ignored such findings, but they encourage treatments which are questionable. In 1987, Dr. Vincent DeVita, Jr., the head of the National Cancer Institute (NCI) from 1980 to 1988, "issued a controversial recommendation to 13,000 cancer specialists in North America to give chemotherapy and surgery to all women with breast cancer, regardless of whether it has spread."[11]

DeVita was a chemotherapy specialist. As such, he conveniently ignored the evidence against his specialty.

There were lots of facts which ought to have gotten in the way of 13,000 cancer specialists recommending to millions of women, "on the highest medical authority," that chemotherapy was needed and in their best interest. Dr. Alan Levin of the University of California San Francisco put the argument against DeVita bluntly:

> "Most cancer patients in this country die of chemotherapy. . . . Chemotherapy does not eliminate breast, colon or lung cancers. The fact has been documented for over a decade. Yet doctors still use chemotherapy for these tumors. . . . Women with breast cancer are likely to die faster with chemotherapy than without it."[12]

British doctor Dick Richards agreed with California doctor Levin. The following statements of Dr. Richards introduce the subject of the criminal culpability of the director of the National Cancer Institute:

> "The real truth is that the orthodox treatment of cancer of the breast in the year 1980 offers no significantly better chance of survival than it did in the year 1900 . . .
>
> "I challenge anyone to show sound evidence that, for example, a random group of advanced breast tumor patients do better when considered as a whole, or even live longer, on surgery, deep x-ray, and chemotherapy, than they do when left totally untreated. In my experience they don't."[13]

In November 1985, Dr. John Cairns of the Harvard School of Public Health, wrote in *Scientific American* that chemotherapy was useful for only a few rare cancers. Dr. Cairns found no significant gains against the primary cancers

10

since the 1950s. He estimated that of the almost 1/2 million Americans who die of cancer each year, only 2% to 3% were being saved by chemotherapy treatment! Dr. Cairns wrote:

"It remains a depressing truth that fewer than 50% of cancer patients can be cured by surgery. . . . It is not possible to detect any sudden change in death rates for any of the major cancers that could be credited to chemotherapy. . . . Those who organize cancer centers and supervise the many clinical trials of chemotherapy look for ways to circumvent these relentless statistics. . . . A six- or twelve-month course of chemotherapy not only is a very unpleasant experience but also has its own intrinsic mortality . . . treatments now avert . . . perhaps 2 or 3 percent . . . of the 400,000 deaths from cancer that occur each year in the U.S."[14]

That is a statistic, which, if widely publicized, would close the cancer treatment centers and force an admission of medical and moral bankruptcy. It also would create an unstoppable public furor in favor of alternative approaches and patient choice. That obviously cannot be permitted by the physicians, researchers, hospitals, drug firms and medical technology companies who benefit so lucratively from the existing system. And the politicians responsible for overseeing such corruption and failure would also catch the wrath of a revengeful public. Remember, we are not talking merely of corruption and incompetence happening somewhere else. We are talking about organized, bureaucratic murder—pain, incalculable suffering and torture happening and having happened to friends and loved ones.

So the newspapers and television do not discuss that damning statistic: 2% to 3% of cancer patients saved by chemotherapy. Instead, DeVita and his co-conspirators recommend chemotherapy and surgery for all breast cancers. The in-depth studies of the worthlessness of surgery, chemotherapy and radiation are not published. The few printed criticisms are one-day news items on back pages which have no impact on cancer treatment and do nothing to spur research into alternative methods.

Meanwhile, millions continue dying while this fascistic nightmare unfolds—and I use the word fascistic purposely

11

because it is the most accurate term, directly linking the modern cancer authorities with their fellow criminals who conducted the medical experiments in Hitler's Germany and Tojo's Japan.

In 1977, Congressional hearings were held on the nation's cancer program. The report concluded that "the public has been misled by the major cancer organizations . . . for the past 25 years." It recommended that those benefiting from the system not be allowed to dictate the choices available to the American public. The Congressional study was ignored. The criminals continue to practice their grisly racket.

In 1984, UCLA doctors Robert Oye and Martin Shapiro exposed one of the gimmicks which the cancer mafia has long used to keep its lethal racket going. Writing in the *Journal of the American Medical Association (JAMA)*, doctors Oye and Shapiro questioned one of the "dirty little secrets." They described how cancer patients were treated with chemotherapy when no evidence existed that the drug would have any effect on their tumors. And they revealed that the new drugs which a physician recommended to a cancer patient were often based on biased studies. False reporting, rigged statistics and exaggerated conclusions were practiced regularly in order to get new drugs approved.[15]

What happens is that patients who die during treatment *are not counted*. Thus the percentage of both those who respond to the drug and those who show no adverse reactions are increased. The dead are not counted—those who not only didn't respond to the new drug, but whose reaction to the drug might have to be designated "fatal." Can't have too many of those. By dying during treatment and sometimes afterward, but in such a way that the drug's effect can't be determined, they often aren't counted.

Here is how the numbers game is played, according to "A Report on Cancer" by Hardin Jones:

> "All reported studies pick up cases at the time of origin of the disease and follow them to death or the end of the study interval. If persons in the untreated or control group die at any time in the study interval, they are reported as deaths in the control group. In the treated group, however, deaths which

occur before completion of treatment are rejected from the data, since these patients do not then meet the criteria established by definition of the term 'treated.' The longer it takes for completion of the treatment, as in multiple step therapy, for example, the worse the error."[9]

In 1986, Dr. John Bailar of Harvard punched another hole in the wall of the cancer industry. Dr. Bailar was a former editor of the journal of the U.S. government's National Cancer Institute (NCI). From this position, he had access to the best statistics and the most advanced scientific basis for modern treatment. An expert in statistical evaluation and statistics consultant to the New England Journal of Medicine as well as senior scientist of the U.S. Department of Health and Human Services's Office of Disease Prevention and Health Promotion, Dr. Bailar had the experience and was in a position to analyze the numbers in such a way as to separate the phony "improvement claims" from the real thing.

In an article he co-authored with Elaine M. Smith from the University of Iowa, Dr. Bailar declared, "We are losing the war against cancer." The controversial article appeared in the May 1986 issue of the prestigious *New England Journal of Medicine*. Bailar and Smith discovered an 8% increase in cancer since 1950, which was steadily worsening. They concluded that "some 35 years of intense effort focused largely on improving treatment must be judged a qualified failure." Regarding breast cancer, they flatly stated, "There has been no apparent change in mortality from breast cancer among white or nonwhite women since 1950."[16]

This kind of objective evaluation had to be contradicted by those in power. So it was. National Cancer Institute leaders, American Cancer Society officials and other interested persons and institutions fired up their propaganda machines. "Cancer statistics indicated great progress," they lied. The reality, which countless hard-eyed citizens could recognize from Bailar and Smith's article, was that a leading expert had "blown the whistle" and that the war on cancer was a failure. But these same hard-eyed citizens who recognized what was being said, especially those at the top of the business, political and media world, were not naïve. They understood that the huge

13

financial incentives to those running the cancer industry made a major course change for the nation almost impossible unless significant leadership emerged to force it.

Nevertheless, Bailar and Smith's report was a milestone. If a significant proportion of the public became aroused or if the few who set the course for society started to recognize an imminent danger to the long-term interest of the nation, furious changes would come—hard and fast. It was too early for such a scenario, but just as the fuse for the Civil War had been lit in "Bleeding Kansas" in the mid-1850s, not exploding until Lincoln's arrival in 1861, so a fuse had been lit in 1986. For the detonation to go off required a celebrity media figure, political leader, economic baron or mass anger to force the issue into the open. America still waits, but the time bomb is ticking.

In 1987, the General Accounting Office, an agency of the U.S. Congress, completed a two-year study of cancer statistics. The results validated Bailar and Smith's conclusions. According to the GAO, $2 billion a year was spent on cancer research, more than half of it being U.S. government funds. Yet, *in all major areas,* only "moderate or slight improvement" in patient survival was indicated for the *three decade* period 1950-1982!

The cancer authorities had lied. Bailar and Smith, Cairns, Levin, Richards and the slowly growing army of opponents to the cancer industry were right. A vast conspiracy of self-interested physicians, hospitals, researchers, bureaucrats, public relations experts and financial corporations were getting rich while millions were being unnecessarily tortured, mutilated and killed.

But the GAO study was argued away, ignored and put on the shelf. The National Cancer Institute's Director, Dr. DeVita, could call for surgery and chemotherapy for all women with breast cancer and no media or political outrage followed. Judy Woodruff of National Education Television's McNeil-Lehr Report could interview Dr. DeVita in 1988 and let him continue making his outrageous claims without a murmur of protest. When letters from informed opponents were received, the show's producers claimed that "they were objective." End of discussion. The monster was still too strong to attack frontally.

How could this be? The stinking, obvious cesspool existed and could be easily documented, yet raising an alarm was like trying to keep the sun from rising. The reporters who were supposed to be the public's voice and early warning system protected the monster. There wasn't a whimper from candidates running for public office. Why? How did the monster become so powerful? How could so much blood and money feed the monster and still no outrage, no courageous backlash from the public or its supposed defenders?

## Chapter two

# The FDA

*"People think the FDA is protecting them—it isn't. What the FDA is doing and what people think it's doing are as different as night and day."*

Herbert L. Ley, Jr., M. D., former
Commissioner of the FDA[17]

*"The hearings have revealed police state tactics . . . possibly perjured testimony to gain a conviction . . . intimidation and gross disregard for Constitutional Rights."*

Senator Edward Long, U.S. Senate
hearings on the FDA[17]

The cancer conspiracy is led by the FDA-NCI-AMA-ACS hierarchy. The initials stand for the Food and Drug Administration (FDA), the National Cancer Institute (NCI), the American Medical Association (AMA), and the American Cancer Society (ACS). The cancer conspiracy also includes the large pharmaceutical companies and key research centers such as the Memorial Sloan-Kettering Cancer Center in New York City and selected university research labs. The key personnel move in and out of official positions within these organizations, sit on common boards or investigation committees, and have both formal and informal networks. When a researcher or alternative medicine advocate is identified as a threat to the power or even the official views put out by the ruling hierarchy, the maverick is placed on various published and unpublished blacklists. Funding is stopped, legal harassment often begins, public denunciation as a quack frequently follows, and if the outsider persists in offering or advocating a non-sanctioned treatment, then rougher, clandestine methods can be employed.

It would take thousands of pages to describe various individuals who have fought the cancer conspiracy and how their threat to the ruling powers was neutralized. These pages can only summarize some of the more famous cases and facts which reveal how the cancer conspiracy functions, but those who wish to know more can pursue the details on their own, using the names and references offered here as a starting point. The people and procedures described in these pages are by no means inclusive, only the most notable or most promising.

The FDA (Food and Drug Administration) is the government police force which approves experimental studies for those it favors and hinders approval for those it dislikes. It conducts semi-legal break-ins (constitutional procedures are often ignored), confiscates records so that critical documentation is often lost or at least unavailable for months and years, and at times has interfered with constitutional protections through conspiratorial relationships with private organizations who share the same suppressive goals. New medical breakthroughs that threaten the sanctioned and financially lucrative treatments are ignored or "studied" for years. The FDA thus frequently subverts its legislated purpose which is to promote and protect the public health. Having lived in Washington, D.C., I know that the FDA is regarded by many astute civil servants as the federal agency with the lowest morale. A dark cloud of oppressive inertia, corruption and bureaucratic sloth pervades its corridors.

Dr. J. Richard Crout, test director at the FDA Bureau of Drugs beginning in 1971, described the agency's agony in Congressional testimony on April 19, 1976 as follows:

> "There was open drunkenness by several employees which went on for months . . . crippled by what some people called the worst personnel in government. There was intimidation internally by people. . . . People, I'm talking about division directors and their staff, would engage in a kind of behavior that invited . . . insubordination—people tittering in corners, throwing spitballs; I am describing physicians, people who would . . . slouch down in a chair, not respond to questions,

moan and groan with sweeping gestures, a kind of behavior I have not seen in any other institution as a grown man. . . . Prior to 1974, not one scientific officer in our place knew his work assignments, nor did any manager know the work assignment of the people under him."[18]

In 1967, FDA stopped the use of an experimental cancer vaccine which was producing significant results. It was developed by H. James Rand, inventor of the heart defibrilator. J. Ernest Ayre, an internationally recognized cancer specialist (co-developer of the PAP test) and Dr. Norbert Czajkowski of Detroit, Michigan assisted Rand. Treating only terminal cancer patients, the Rand vaccine produced objective improvement in 35% of 600 patients while another 30% demonstrated subjective improvement. "One 65 year old woman with spreading tumor" was "completely cured in 4 months." Another woman with extensive breast cancer was cured in 6 months. The FDA stopped the vaccine's use in a federal court hearing where neither the cancer patients *nor their doctors* were allowed to testify. When U.S. Senator Stephen Young of Ohio protested, it was to no avail. Senator Young could get nowhere with FDA Commissioner James L. Goddard. Senator Young recalled:

"I could not move them. They would not even agree to a modification of the ruling (banning the Rand vaccine), which would at least allow the 100 (cancer) patients at Richmond Heights (Ohio) to complete their injections. The Justice Department was prepared to go along, but the FDA Commissioner, Dr. James Goddard, was adamant, even belligerent. It's wrong of the government to snatch away this hope when there is no evidence against its use offered in court. It's damnably wrong."[19]

It is known that when FDA Commissioner Goddard's own wife had serious health problems and orthodox medicine could not help her, Goddard contacted alternative health practitioners who quietly healed his wife. But for the suffering victims of cancer who needed the Rand vaccine or some other non-traditional treatment, Goddard lowered the boom, using the federal courts to enforce his dictum. Such are the ways of the FDA.

Goddard's greatest disservice to the American people was his persecution of DMSO, a simple molecule which often brought miraculous pain relief and offered numerous possibilities for medical advancement in other areas, including cancer. One respected science writer suggested that Goddard crushed DMSO research in order to gain increased police powers from Congress. The FDA has never admitted its errors regarding DMSO although the positive studies from qualified scientists number over a thousand while the FDA's criticisms have been shown to be almost completely based on lies or unsubstantiated rumors. Yet by the late 1980s, twenty years later, the FDA continues to imprison DMSO advocates. The malignity of Goddard's arbitrary and conscienceless acts in 1966-1968 against reputable scientists, dedicated doctors and the public good is one of the darkest chapters of FDA history.

No one is sure of the real reasons why it happened and why it continues to be covered up twenty years later. It has been suggested that one or more drug companies sabotaged DMSO because it threatened so many of their profitable products. One drug company executive reportedly told the leading DMSO researcher:

"I don't care if it is the major drug of our century—and we all know it is—it isn't worth it to us."[20]

Who had the power to keep such a miraculous drug off the shelves? Surely not just an FDA Commissioner flexing his muscle. Was it a combination of drug companies whose individual profits were threatened by the miracle drug's possibilities?

"(It is) not our (FDA) policy to jeopardize the financial interests of the pharmaceutical companies."

from testimony before Congress of
Dr. Charles C. Edwards, at the
time Commissioner of the FDA[21]

It has also been surmised that FDA Commissioner Goddard used DMSO in 1966 in an attempt to become the medical dictator of America. In the years that followed, FDA officials simply refused to expose the agency's "dirty laundry." Hence the on-going suppression of what many recognize as "the major drug of the century."

In any case, Goddard instilled fear into honest researchers and physicians as no previous FDA Commissioner had done. He ruined careers. He introduced an intensified police force mentality into FDA with his emphasis on hiring ex T-men and G-men. He consciously blacklisted scientists as punishment for opposing him. And members of his agency, either with his encouragement or his acquiescence, openly began ignoring the Constitution for the sake of promotions and power.

Pat McGrady, Sr.'s book, *The Persecuted Drug: The Story of DMSO,* detailed what Goddard's FDA did. McGrady described "the no-knock system, the photocopying of private papers, bugging, punitive investigations, slander and libel, character assassination, forgery, lying and blackmail."[22]

One scientist declared to McGrady:

"For the first time in my life I know fear. I'm afraid for my family and myself. I'm afraid for doctors and scientists. And I'm more afraid for our country. I can't believe these things are happening in the United States."

Another noted researcher maligned by Goddard's FDA observed:

"The academic community and industry are so completely intimidated that one cannot look for any leadership to counteract some of the punitive actions of the FDA. . . . I am very pessimistic concerning the future status of medical research unless a mood arises to combat overzealous bureaucratic authority."

Dr. Walter Modell of Cornell University Medical College finally warned in a published article ("FDA Censorship" in *Clinical Pharmacology and Therapeutics*):

"When the nonexpert ingroup of the FDA threatens to become the dictator of American medicine we believe it will lead medicine from its respected eminence to its ultimate decline."[22]

A few years after the DMSO suppression, one of Goddard's top aides, Billy Goodrich, left the FDA with his pension and became president of a food association regulated by the FDA. A personal friend who had been president of the food association took over Billy Goodrich's position at FDA. They simply switched jobs! Congressmen screamed in protest. It was such a blatant demonstration of the "musical shuffle" (which Congress had previously observed but ignored) that they *had* to make noise this time in order to avert public wrath. Still, after all the sound and fury, nothing happened.

Goddard himself became Chairman of the Board of Ormont Drug and Chemical Company a few years after leaving FDA.

A study conducted by the U.S. Congress in 1969 revealed that 37 of 49 top officials of the FDA who left the agency moved into high corporate positions with the large companies they had regulated. A General Accounting Office (GAO) study of FDA in 1975 revealed that 150 FDA officials owned stock in the companies they were supposed to regulate. The record of "conflict of interest" (or worse) within the FDA is deep and extensive.

In 1976, Dr. J. Richard Crout of the FDA admitted that "endless questions" was a favored technique within the agency to discourage any researcher who sought approval for an unorthodox cancer therapy. Bureaucratic obstruction is a weapon as deadly as a gun when the lives of innocent millions are at stake. It is a delusion to consider such institutionalized, orchestrated conduct, consciously chosen either because of orders from above or personal inclination, as anything other than white collar murder. It closely resembles the role carried out by the bureaucrats who pushed the paper in Nazi Germany. The policymakers may not fully perceive the effect of their actions, but the horror has gone on for too many decades to allow a plea of ignorance to be totally convincing.

In 1972, Dean Burk, Ph.D. of the National Cancer Institute (head of their cytochemistry section and a veteran of 32 years at the agency) declared in a letter to a member of Congress that high officials of the FDA, AMA, ACS and the U.S. Department of Health, Education and Welfare (now Health and Human Services or HHS) were deliberately falsifying information, literally lying, committing unconstitutional acts and in other ways thwarting potential cancer cures to which they were opposed.

Dr. Burk's famous May 30, 1972 letter to Congressman Louis Frey, Jr. dealt with the issue of why FDA had revoked an Investigative New Drug (IND) application. The IND application, according to Dr. Burk, was superior to many routinely approved. But it involved testing laetrile, a controversial, non-patentable product opposed by the California Medical Association (CMA). FDA approved the original application, then rescinded the license, apparently because of pressure from the surgeon general, a member of the CMA and a laetrile foe.

Dr. Burk was not an advocate of laetrile. He was however in favor of fair testing. He was totally opposed to what he bluntly called "misleading and indeed fraudulent" FDA reports. In his correspondence with Congress, he openly referred to the "FDA corruption."

Corruption indeed. It takes several forms. Refusing to allow investigation of a non-toxic compound which might help cancer patients is one. Failing to assert itself when a drug tested on human beings was determined to cause cancer is another. Here are the facts of such a case:

In August 1969 it was learned that a drug called Cinanserin, produced by E. R. Squibb and Sons, Princeton, New Jersey, caused tumors in the livers of rats. Human testing of the drug was thus stopped. But Squibb's executives did not want to do follow-ups on the humans who had taken Cinanserim.

For three years, FDA tried to *persuade* Squibb to do follow-up studies. (Compare this approach with what FDA does to alternative cancer treatments which work—raids, confiscation of documents, jail, etc. With the large drug companies, FDA tries persuasion!)

Finally, in 1972, FDA and the National Academy of Sciences set up a committee to examine procedures on follow-ups when a drug was found to be dangerous. Who was appointed to head the committee? The vice-president of Squibb whom the FDA had tried for 3 years to persuade to do follow-ups on those people who had been given the cancer-causing drug![23]

FDA has a long history of ignoring dangerous drugs and chemical additives marketed by the big drug companies while using bureaucratic delays, legal harassment, unconstitutional procedures, and even falsified evidence to stop unorthodox cancer treatments. In 1964, FDA inititated a multimillion dollar prosecution of Andrew Ivy, Vice-President and professor of physiology at the University of Illinois. Ivy was former chairman of the National Cancer Institute's National Advisory Council on Cancer. He was an internationally recognized scholar and a prolific author of scientific papers.

His sin was that he supported a cancer-curing serum called Krebiozen. Over 20,000 cancer patients had supposedly benefited from Krebiozen. One United States Senate Committee lawyer personally assessed 530 cases and concluded that Krebiozen was effective.

Among the doctors who supported it was US Air Force Major General Wallace H. Graham, Physician to the President of the United States:

> "I have had some . . . unusually good results with Krebiozen."[7]

It made no difference.

According to David Rorvik:

> "Despite the government's (FDA's) multi-million dollar prosecution, which lasted 289 days and included falsified testimony, later confessed by the government, the four defendants (including Ivy) were acquitted on all 240 counts brought against them. The jury went to the extraordinary length, moreover, of saying that it believed Krebiozen had merit and should be tested, on the basis of positive, often well-documented testimony it had heard."[3]

Krebiozen has never been tested objectively. FDA used illegal methods to stop it, methods which have been part of a conscious goal at FDA to dictate what medicine a citizen is permitted to use and what he may not use. Combined with the questionable behavior of FDA officials, the stock links to the large drug companies, and the testimony of FDA employees that conscious cover-ups were common, the intention of FDA to dictate individual medicine has to be recognized as one of the most dangerous threats to freedom that has ever existed.

Peter Temin, a professor at MIT, carefully studied FDA history and policy for his 1980 book, *Taking Your Medicine: Drug Regulation in the United States*. His conclusion, based on a very careful, close look at FDA is frightening:

> "The most important facet of FDA regulation is the agency's expression of its conviction that individuals—both doctors and consumers—cannot make reasonable choices among drugs.

"The agency tried with increasing success to deny drug pre-
scribers and users the option of taking 'innocuous' drugs, that
is, to force them to use drugs the FDA regards as appropriate
for their condition."[24]

Despite evidence which extends for decades, revealing
criminal behavior in the one agency that holds the power to
permit tests of alternative cures for cancer, Congress has done
nothing. One night in Washington, D.C., I found out why. I
was introduced to the aide of one of the most powerful U.S.
Representatives in Congress. His boss had been in Washington
for many years. Yet, despite the Congressman's powerful
committee position and ranking status in the majority party,
he was unable to do anything with the health officials at FDA
or NCI. After a number of drinks, this Congressman's aide
told me that FDA and NCI were protected fiefdoms. They
wrote their own legislation, permitting only minor changes by
Congress. They ignored Congressional complaints. They were
extensively tied to the big drug companies. They "know no
one controls them. No one is able to take a sword and tell
them where to go," the aide said. He leaned across the table
and whispered, "Only national security procedures are as
tightly controlled, without outside examination. Only national
security. Does that tell you something?"

It told me that the monster was real and dangerous if some
of the most powerful men in the U.S. Congress, with their
massive egos and independent political bases, were afraid of
it.

G. E. Griffin, author of *World Without Cancer,* made
explicit the fundamental, systematic wrong which has emerged
out of the various crosscurrents that make up FDA—underpaid
civil servants playing it safe, drug companies and their
Washington lawyers putting unending pressure on the bureaucrats, academic medicos controlling the approval process and
restricting the individual doctor's choice, revolving door
employment between FDA and universities/drug companies,
and behind-the-scenes political deals. According to Griffin,
FDA did two things: (1) they "protected" the big drug companies and were subsequently rewarded; and (2) they
attacked—using the government's police powers—those who
threatened the big drug companies, be it a young company

25

with a new product, a breakthrough miracle drug such as DMSO, or natural health store products such as food, vitamins, minerals or other self-healing (non-drug, non-doctor) methods.

Griffin wrote the following about FDA:

"First, it is providing a means whereby key individuals on its payroll are able to obtain both power and wealth through granting special favors to certain politically influential groups that are subject to its regulation. This activity is similar to the 'protection racket' of organized crime: for a price, one can induce FDA administrators to provide 'protection' from the FDA itself.

"Secondly, as a result of this political favoritism, the FDA has become a primary factor in that formula whereby cartel-oriented companies in the food and drug industry are able to use the police powers of government to harass or destroy their free-market competitors.

"And thirdly, the FDA occasionally does some genuine public good with whatever energies it has left over after serving the vested political and commercial interest of its first two activities."[7]

There is only one solution. No reform will work. REPEAT: NO REFORM WILL WORK. No changing of personnel will have any long term effect. No new laws dealing with regulations. Only one solution.

It was provided by a southern doctor now living in New York City who has observed the monster in action for many years. Raymond Keith Brown, M.D. outlined the solution in his book, *Cancer, AIDS and the Medical Establishment*. He described how the power which FDA has to approve drugs and technology has to be eliminated and replaced with the solitary role of testing for effectiveness and safety, the results being the basis for FDA labeling. The *individual physician* and *individual patient* would regain the responsibility to use or not use a given drug or technology.

Dr. Brown recommended:

"The FDA should follow a simple rating system for effectiveness and safety. Effectiveness would fall into one of three categories 'Effectiveness Unconditionally Proved', 'Effectiveness Conditionally Demonstrated', and 'Effectiveness Undetermined.' Safety could also be categorized in the same manner and the appropriate designation then affixed to all products or containers. Judgment of the effectiveness of any medical product or device should not be vested in any governmental agency or institutions, but should be returned to the province of the individual physician. Freedom of choice for medical materials, therapy and methods must be put on the same footing as civil liberties and as vigorously protected."[25]

One of the better scholars in this field—Robert G. Houston—says simply:

"There should be curbs on the FDA—on its powers to intrude into the private practice of medicine . . . FDA should not be dictating to doctors what they can and cannot do."[26]

Richard Ericson, a dedicated husband of a cancer victim, eloquently concurred (*Cancer Treatment: Why So Many Failures?*):

"A physician should be able to prescribe any type of cancer treatment that he considers best for the patient, with the patient's consent and knowledge, without stringent governmental regulations that are now in force. Congress should consider such problems when new guidelines are enacted."

Only when FDA concentrates on the blatant health menaces such as overtly misleading health product claims or drugs shown to cause death and injury; only when FDA ceases to be the bully boy for the big drug companies and other vested interests; and only when FDA again allows physicians, nonconventional healers and their patients some choice of therapeutic treatments . . . will it regain its legitimate government function. In its present form, it is like a malignant beast harming society rather than serving it.

Chapter Three

# The AMA

*"The essence of modern dictatorship is the combination of one-dimensional, flat thinking with power and terror."*

Theodore Haecker[27]

The American Medical Association (AMA) has a long history of corruption. Its most infamous leader was Morris Fishbein who reigned from 1924 until 1949. He had failed anatomy in medical school and had never practiced medicine a day in his life, but during his years in power he was recognized as the virtual dictator of American medicine. Journalist and scholar Ruth Mulvey Harmer, Ph.D. characterized Fishbein as having the "ruthlessness of a shark" and concluded that he "managed to hold back the twentieth century for 50 years for the benefit of organized medicine" (*American Medical Avarice*, 1975).

Those who paid large advertising sums to the AMA Journal were given the AMA "seal of approval" for their products, despite the lack of any benefit, while those who wouldn't pay the advertising tax often had their products labeled as worthless. It was essentially a lucrative blackmail scheme.

Fishbein supported drugs but adamantly opposed any food or natural remedies.

Fishbein's opposition to any therapy or technology unrelated to drugs was based on the simple fact that the AMA's power base and economic growth *required* drug sales. Anything which threatened the growing dependency on drugs threatened the AMA's entire empire. Public health was not and could not be the primary concern of the AMA. Pulitzer Prize (1984) author Paul Starr explained the interlocking interests in his award-winning book, *The Social Transformation of American Medicine:*

> "Medical authority in prescribing drugs and other products enabled the AMA to stand between the manufacturers and their markets. This strategic gatekeeping role permitted the AMA, in effect, to levy an advertising toll on the producers. Revenues from journal advertisements became the principal source of funds for the association. In 1912 the AMA set up a cooperative advertising bureau, which channeled advertisements to state medical journals. The bureau gave the AMA considerable financial leverage over the state medical societies and helped bind the national association even more tightly together."[28]

Evidence cited by Eustace Mullins in his 1988 book, *Murder by Injection,* suggests that Fishbein ignored medical documentation to the effect that products promoted by the AMA were dangerous. According to Mullins, one such product caused blindness in a number of people. Another quietly killed people in their sleep. Another was so poisonous that it eventually caused the deaths of many, many people.

Another of Fishbein's primary interests was his attempt to corner the rights on promising cancer treatments, or insure that any cancer treatment which threatened AMA financial interests was kept from the public. When the owners of a promising cancer treatment refused to sell it to the AMA, "difficulties" started.

In collaboration with the government and private interests within the cancer industry, Fishbein and his successors have left a history of illegal acts, bribery, conspiracy against medical innovation, monopolistic suppression of competitors and contributing to the physical mutilation and death of patients and consumers.

In the 1930s, a California researcher named Royal R. Rife developed a bio-electronic instrument which destoryed various viruses in a non-invasive, painless treatment. In association with the University of Southern California, a number of clinics used Rife's technology to cure terminal cancer during the period 1934-38. Some of the leading researchers in the country and leading physicians in Southern California participated. In

1938, the AMA's Fishbein found out about the Rife cancer cure and tried to "buy in." When the offer was refused, the entire program was destroyed within six months. First all the doctors were visited and told to abandon the instrument or they would lose their medical licenses and go to jail. Then the leading medical electronic laboratory in America, where Rife's treatment was being independently validated, was burned to the ground at 3 A.M. in the morning while its director was in California consulting with Rife. Three months later, Rife was hauled into court and the treatment was effectively quashed.

This was not the only occasion when scientists or doctors who opposed the AMA or whose discoveries threatened the AMA's financial gains were "burned out," or arrested on trumped-up charges, or died mysteriously. Howard Beard, Ph.D., Director of Biochemistry at LSU Medical School and developer of a urine test for determining cancer, recalled:

> "Early one morning in 1946, our lab was mysteriously destroyed by fire. . . . We then established a lab at our present location. Then again one morning in 1947 this lab was set on fire and completely destroyed."[29]

Dr. William F. Koch, the inventor of Glyoxylide, was a particular target of Fishbein and the AMA. So were the doctors who supported him and used the cancer serum Dr. Koch invented.

> "One doctor . . . J. W. Kannel, saved a young girl. . . . She had hopeless cancer of the spleen. . . . One shot of Glyoxylide, and she became well (in 1943 and was still alive in 1983). . . . Kannel was barred from all hospitals in Fort Wayne."[30]

> "One death from poisoning, and one from being run down by an automobile, both victims being physicians of distinction and prominent in the advocacy of the Koch treatment. . . . Dr. Koch himself was the target of at least 13 unsuccessful attempts on his life."[31]

Fishbein and his associates at the AMA had been interested in the Harry Hoxsey cancer treatment since 1924. In that year, Dr. Malcolm Harris, the chief surgeon at two Chicago hospitals and later President of the AMA, offered to purchase the Hoxsey cancer tonic. Hoxsey would get 10% of the profits after ten years! The AMA doctors would set the fees and keep all the profits for the first nine years and 90% of the profits from the tenth year. When Hoxsey refused the offer of Dr. Harris, Fishbein began years of official intimidation. Doctors who worked with Hoxsey lost their licenses. Pathologists who examined tumors for Hoxsey lost their businesses. State medical boards closed free clinics where hundreds of "terminal" cancer patients were being saved.

In Iowa, Hoxsey was treating 300 patients a day in the late 1920s. During the vicious 1937-39 period when Fishbein was stopping Rife's treatment, Hoxsey was charged more than a hundred times with practicing medicine without a license in Texas.

Still, Hoxsey's Dallas clinic grew to the point where it was handling as many as 12,000 patients, with affiliate clinics being established in Illinois, Pennsylvania and other states. In a legal action against Fishbein and the AMA in 1949, Hoxsey won. Fishbein's attorney admitted that Hoxsey's treatment did cure cancer. Judge W. L. Thorton ruled:

> "I am of the firm opinion and belief that Hoxsey has cured these people of cancer. Hoxsey has been done a great injustice and . . . articles and utterances by defendant Morris Fishbein were false, slanderous, and libelous."

Nevertheless, through an organized conspiracy of the AMA, the FDA and the NCI, Hoxsey's clinics were closed. His treatments have never been officially tested, despite admissions by opponents that they work and court testimony by experts which resulted in a jury concluding that Hoxsey's cancer treatment had therapeutic value. Hoxsey's primary assistant still operates a Hoxsey clinic in Mexico.[32]

A documentary film on Hoxsey is available.[33]

In 1946, Fishbein initiated an attack against Dr. Max Gerson, whose dietary treatments for cancer were anathema to the drug and business-oriented Fishbein. The laboratories used by Dr. Gerson were later threatened with economic ruin if they continued to provide services to him. His diet, so vehemently opposed by the AMA in 1946, now closely resembles the anti-cancer diets recommended by the orthodox cancer organizations in the 1980s.[34]

Attempts against Gerson's life also were made:

> "On two occasions Gerson became violently ill. . . . Lab tests showed . . . arsenic in his urine. Some of Gerson's best case histories mysteriously disappeared from his files. The manuscript and all its copies for Gerson's almost completed book were stolen and never recovered."[35]

In 1946, a Senate subcommittee heard testimony from cancer patients successfully treated by Dr. Gerson. The Senator in charge was Claude Pepper of Florida. When he initiated legislation to conquer cancer, the AMA turned its power against Senator Pepper. He was defeated for re-election to the Senate. Pepper later returned to the U.S. Congress as a representative, but ever afterward *served* orthodox medical interests. He had learned his lesson. Until his death in 1989, he was the leading promoter of "quack investigations" for orthodox medicine, writing to the various state attorneys general for assistance in quashing different alternative treatments. As a national celebrity and "staunch defender" of older Americans, he was the perfect front man for the medical and drug cartels. He was more like a Judas to the elderly, but history alone will assess Claude Pepper's true infamy. Like many men, he ignored the deaths of millions of people for the sake of his own well-being and political position.

In 1953, U.S. Senator Charles Tobey began a Senate investigation into the cancer industry. Attorney Ben Fitzgerald of the U.S. Justice Department was hired as special counsel to the Senate Interstate and Foreign Commerce Committee to lead the investigation. Fitzgerald's final report concluded that the AMA, in collaboration with the NCI and FDA, entered into a conspiracy to suppress alternative, effective cancer treatments. The August 28, 1953 Congressional Record contained the following summary of special counsel Fitzgerald:

> "There is reason to believe that the AMA has been hasty, capricious, arbitary, and outright dishonest . . .
> "If radium, X-ray or surgery or either of them is the com-

plete answer, then the greatest hoax of the age is being perpetrated upon the people by the continued appeal for funds for further research. If neither X-ray, radium or surgery is the complete answer to this dreaded disease, and I submit that it is not, then what is the plain duty of society? Should we stand still? Should we sit idly by and count the number of physicians, surgeons and cancerologists who are not only divided but who, because of fear or favor, are forced to line up with the so-called accepted view of the American Medical Association, or should this Committee make a full-scale investigation of the organized effort to hinder, suppress and restrict the free flow of drugs which allegedly have proven successful in cases where clinical records, case history, pathological reports and X-ray photographic proof, together with the alleged cured patients, are available?

"Accordingly, we should determine whether existing agencies, both public and private, are engaged in and have pursued a policy of harassment, ridicule, slander and libelous attacks on others sincerely engaged in stamping out this curse of mankind. Have medical associations, through their officers, agents, servants and employees engaged in this practice? My investigation to date should convince this Committee that a conspiracy does exist to stop the free flow and use of drugs in interstate commerce which allegedly (have) solid therapeutic value. Public and private funds have been thrown around like confetti at a country fair to close up and destroy clinics, hospitals, and scientific research laboratories which do not conform to the viewpoint of medical associations. How long will the American people take this?"[2]

That report of the United States Congress was issued over 35 years ago. The conspiracy has continued, grown stronger, and in many ways is more ruthless today. Senator Tobey soon conveniently died of a heart attack. (This has happened to others who were in a position to threaten the cancer industry.) The man who replaced Senator Tobey as head of the Committee was Senator John Bricker, who had been a lawyer for several drug companies. His first act was to order Ben Fitzgerald to stop the investigation into the cancer conspiracy. Fitzgerald refused and was fired. Thus ended the first major national investigation into the criminal conspiracy between the government's health agencies and private medical organizations to monopolize cancer treatment.

34

In researching the book on Royal Rife's 1934 cure for cancer\*, I discovered several doctors who had practiced in the 1940s and 1950s. They told tales of office break-ins, telephone wiretaps and other kinds of harassment that happened to physicians who opposed the AMA or even advocated therapies which the AMA considered financially threatening. One physician who talked on the radio against the AMA was beaten several times, the thugs waiting outside the radio stations when he finished. Another had to be escorted to the Mexican border by his armed brother, so terrified was he of reprisals. Much of the darker side of the AMA's efforts will never be known, now lost to history, but pieces suggest some very dirty tactics were used while law officials looked the other way.

In 1971, the AMA's Council on Drugs, an independent group of scientists and doctors, completed a $3 million evaluation on prescription drugs. Over 300 experts had been involved. Unfortunately, Max H. Parrott, chairman of the board of directors of the AMA, did not like what the independent council concluded in regard to drugs. He asked that the report not be published until "our friends" at the Pharmaceutical Manufacturers Association (PMA) looked at it.

The PMA came back with "three or four crates" of revisions, but the independent Council refused to make major changes, especially in its criticism of the drug companies' heavily advertised drug combinations.

In September 1972, a second edition of the "AMA Drug Evaluation" was ready and the Council gave the AMA Board of Directors another advance look. One month later, the AMA disbanded its independent Council on Drugs.

On February 6, 1973, two former chairmen and one vice-chairman of the AMA's Council on Drugs testified before Congress. They accused the AMA of being "a captive of and beholden to the pharmaceutical industry."[23]

The ad revenues from the drug companies, which had been the basis for the AMA's power and had distorted medical procedures and policies for decades, was shown to be still the driving force behind the AMA in the 1970s. It hasn't changed in the 1980s. Policies and procedures which are in the health

\* The Cancer Cure That Worked—see note 67.

35

interest of the public, but not in the financial interest of the drug companies, are suppressed.

In 1987, the AMA was found guilty of conspiring for 20 years to destroy the profession of chiropractic. The court concluded, "Under the Sherman Act, every combination or conspiracy in restraint of trade is illegal. The court has held that the conduct of the AMA and its members constituted a conspiracy in restraint of trade" (September 25, 1987). But nothing halted the far more lethal AMA practice of attacking alternative cancer physicians and alternative practitioners (non MDs) using non-drug approaches, through the state medical licensing boards, district attorneys and business networks.

The AMA consists of less than 300,000 dues-paying members (out of more than 750,000 physicians in the U.S.). It employs approximately 900 people at its Chicago headquarters and another 400 in Washington, D.C. Its 1986 budget was $122 million. Approximately two and a half million dollars goes to Washington, D.C. to oversee its lobbying efforts. In 1986, it budgeted approximately four and one-half million dollars to elect key Congressmen for committees critical in developing medical legislation (or defeating those who opposed the AMA's interests).

A very small number of persons will determine the course of the nation's health in the crisis years ahead. AMA officials, their lobbyists and their Congressmen will be on one side. The other side will consist of the few Congressmen who have consistently fought the AMA for the public's benefit. The public doesn't even know who these secret heroes and heroines are.

A shutting-off of the AMA's power to dictate medical treatment and organize blatant conspiracies that destroy individuals and organizations which attempt to offer alternative treatments for cancer, is long overdue. And the reader should not presume that the suppression of doctors practicing alternative medicine is past history. Robert G. Houston, a noted scholar in the field, has concluded that today's offensives against innovative healers are as bad as ever:

> "There is evidence that this is all coordinated in a massive movement to stamp out all alternative doctors. . . . At least fifty and probably more like a hundred doctors in the past two

36

years have undergone such treatment, called before licensing boards."[26]

A few years ago, the Vice-President of the AMA admitted his organization was nothing but a union. Therefore, perhaps it is appropriate that the public start coldly viewing the AMA doctors as an organized conspiracy in restraint of trade. AMA Vice-President James Sammons stated on the November 22, 1982 Phil Donahue show:

> "Our reasons for being in political action are exactly the same as the AFL-CIO. Exactly."[7]

Perhaps the most powerful of the state organizations affiliated with the AMA is the California Medical Association (CMA). California is a natural hotbed for innovative therapies. Thus the CMA guardian role in keeping alternative therapies restricted is a critical one. If California were to open its doors to alternative therapies (for cancer and otherwise) which successfully provided a viable alternative to the seriously ill patient, the entire national program of the AMA could be threatened.

According to a 1987 article in the *San Diego Union,* the CMA was the largest cash contributor to the state legislators for the previous five years. Most significant, the article reported what the CMA got for its payoff money:

> "that of the 155 bills that the CMA adamantly opposed last year, not a single one was enacted into law by the Legislature."[36]

Two remedies are necessary—(1) setting up alternative medical boards in each state, and (2) recognizing and defending each citizen's freedom to choose any medical treatment without interference from an organized *minority* of doctors. (The AMA membership has included less than half the allopathic doctors in the U.S. since 1971. Now only 40% or so of the nation's allopathic physicians and 0% of alternative practitioners belong to it.)

No nation has any realistic expectation of a better future, especially in a rapidly changing, competitive world, if its health system is corrupt or fundamentally opposed to innovation. Recent comparisons of Americans with Europeans, using sophisticated diagnostic instruments, indicated that Americans were much sicker than their trans-Atlantic cousins. One cause certainly can be traced to the decades of conspiratorial machinations by the AMA in its attempt to own, control or suppress new therapies for cancer and other diseases.

This situation does not have to continue. A citizen's right to a choice between competing health practitioners, including non-MDs (non-drug therapists), has long been recognized in international law, particularly the Nuremberg Code. The principle has even been articulated by an outstanding political leader, Dwight Eisenhower, the AMA's own Judicial Council, and the AMA President. But Federal and State laws must guarantee these rights. Otherwise, organizations such as the AMA will continue to obstruct them through state medical licensing boards and state "medical quality" laws. And these rights must apply to the cancer patient, not just the relatively healthy person who wants to shop for therapies.

"The right of the individual to elect freely the manner of his care in illness must be preserved."

Dwight D. Eisenhower, President
of the United States, 1953-1961

"The freedom of the individual to select his preferred system of medical care and free competition among physicians and alternative systems of medical care are prerequisites of ethical practice and optimal medical care."

Judicial Council of the
AMA, 1981

"The individual's freedom of choice remains a cornerstone of the American system."

Dr. Alan R. Nelson, President,
AMA, March 7, 1990

Chapter Four

# The ACS

*"Cancer is one of the most curable of the major diseases in this country."*

American Cancer Society booklet

*"They (ACS) lie like scoundrels."*

Dean Burk, Ph.D., 34 years at
the National Cancer Institute[37]

The American Cancer Society is one of the most powerful and corrupt organizations in American society. It operates as a behind-the-scenes force, influencing powerful politicians, imposing its views and prejudices on governmental research, instigating government suppression and harassment of independent researchers, making newspaper editors cower, and all the while asking the public for money through its public relations image as the leading cancer fighter. Its key people must bear heavy responsibility for the millions of American lives lost while potential alternative therapies for cancer were "ground under" the ACS's heavy boot.

Formed in 1913, the American Cancer Society was reorganized in 1944 under the leadership of Albert Lasker, an advertising tycoon, and Elmer Bobst, president of two drug companies, Hoffman LaRoche and Warner Lambert. The driving force of the ACS for decades was the dragon lady of the cancer industry, Mary Lasker of New York City. The Albert and Mary Lasker Foundation, based on Albert Lasker's huge fortune from advertising, gave Mary Lasker the clout to dominate cancer research. Albert Lasker's "great" contribution to the world was his Lucky Strike cigarette ads and his campaigns to encourage women to smoke, which included many Hol-

39

lywood films showing women smoking. He was, in my opinion, personally responsible for millions of American women (and women around the world) dying of lung cancer.

After the Laskers took over the American Cancer Society, its board was dominated by representatives from big banks, drug companies and status-quo research organizations. Using its behind-the-scenes political and financial clout, the American Cancer Society can make or break researchers as well as significantly influence, if not determine, the national cancer research agenda.

From its earliest years under the Laskers' direction, ACS has intended to steal public funds for its own use. Albert Lasker died in 1952, only six years after he and Elmer Bobst took over the ACS, but Mary Lasker recalled her husband's advice years later:

> "When I asked my husband for money for the American Cancer Society to do research, he said, 'No, I'm not going to give you any money'—although he did. But he said, 'The place to get money is the federal government.' And I said, 'I don't know anything about the government.' And he said, 'There are unlimited funds. I'll show you how to get them.'"[38]

Mary Lasker did so with a vengeance.

It was in the 1950s that Mary Lasker and her friends laid the foundation for their massive 1970s assault on the U.S. Treasury. According to historian James T. Patterson, "Mary and her Little Lambs" virtually ruled the health agenda of the American nation. Florence Mahoney, a friend of Mary's and the wife of an heir to the Cox newspaper chain, moved to Washington in 1950. She became the "unofficial hostess for the health lobby." From 1952 to 1961, because of the Lasker Lobby, the National Cancer Institute's budget went from $18 million to $110 million. Half of it was absorbed by chemotherapy. It was not a coincidence that Cornelius Rhoads, who was head of the Memorial Sloan-Kettering Cancer Center in New York (and who had been chief medical officer of the Army's Chemical Warfare Division during World War II) pushed chemotherapy hard despite little results. He often appeared in public relations work for the American Cancer Society. He also openly bragged about being the per-

40

son who would cure cancer, while clandestinely interfering with cancer researchers who had different ideas.

Mary Lasker's top Washington lobbyist was Mike Gorman. Gorman boasted that Lasker's network was:

"probably unparalelled in the influence that a small group of private citizens has over such a major area of national policy . . . high class kind of subversion, very high class. We're not second story burglars. We go right in the front door."[39]

By the mid-1950s a few doctors and scientists had recognized what was happening, but the Lasker political steamroller was too strong to stop. Patterson quotes one doctor who complained that the National Cancer Institute was merely:

"a tool of the American Cancer Society, making a propaganda pitch for that organization. . . . They subsidize and perpetuate ignorance and fraud in the mistaken belief that they are benefiting humanity."[39]

By the end of the 1950s, a few Congressmen were also growing suspicious. They saw the money rolling in, the lack of any progress against cancer, and in fact the beginning of the ACS opposition to anyone interfering with their "racket." U.S. Congressman Roland Libonati complained:

"Maybe the raising of millions of dollars of funds for charitable projects has become a 'racket', and the longer they remain in the test-tube stage of development, the longer patronage and job payrollers remain in their soft berths. . . . Maybe we should investigate the American Cancer Society's operations."[7]

Yet the 1950s and 1960s were only a warm-up for the American Cancer Society. The big payoff would be the 1970s.

In 1969, Mary Lasker initiated the "war on cancer" which was signed into law in December 1971 by President Richard Nixon. Nixon's career had been revived by Elmer Bobst, the other power at the ACS, when he arranged for Nixon to be hired at a Wall Street law firm following Nixon's defeat for President in 1960 and defeat for Governor of California in 1962. The war on cancer became a financial bonanza for those favored by the ACS. Because of the enormous public funds available to these pirates, they zealously restricted access to their little kingdom. Outsiders with innovative therapies were not welcomed. Samuel S. Epstein, professor of preventive medicine and community health at the University of Illinois Medical Society in Chicago described how the "war on cancer" began:

"The cancer lobby, headed by the late Sydney Farber, politically astute director of the Children's Cancer Research Foundation, Boston, and including the American Cancer Society and Mary Lasker, a New York philanthropist who had close contacts with the administrations of successive Presidents, exerted a powerful influence on Congress and the public. Both were exhorted by hard-sell techniques (to believe) that the cure for cancer was just around the corner, and only needed more support and funding for the American Cancer Society and NCI. In the naive search for the 'magic bullet,' the NCI financed a huge and ill-conceived Cancer Chemotherapy Program for mass-screening of hundreds of chemicals, selected on tenuous pretexts, for anticancer activity in tissue culture and animal tumor systems."[40]

A full page ad was put in the *New York Times* on December 9, 1969 to start the "war on cancer" campaign. It read, "We are so close to a cure for cancer. We lack only the will and the kind of money and comprehensive planning that went into putting a man on the moon."

Four or five months later, Mary Lasker contacted her friend Mathilde Krim, a research biologist at Memorial Sloan-Kettering Cancer Center and also politically-connected through her friendship with ex-President Lyndon Johnson. Together Lasker and Krim went off to Washington and soon had a Senator interested in the war on cancer. An outside panel, composed mainly of people associated with the American Cancer Society, was assigned to draft a report. Mathilde Krim became fascinated with interferon during her preparation of a major portion of the report.

Once the report was completed, a bill was offered in the Senate. Then the newspaper advice columnist Ann Landers joined the crusade. Soon a public groundswell was created. Many scientists in cancer research were opposed to the notion of billions of dollars going to cancer. They rightly surmised that most of it would be wasted. But Mary Lasker never paid much attention to the scientists. At the end of 1971, President Nixon signed the war on cancer into law. Mary Lasker's public relations campaign had succeeded. Now the public funds were in the water and the sharks moved in for the feast.

Lucy Eisenberg provided the following insights in a November 1971 article in *Harper's*:

> "the so-called Conquest of Cancer Act is the product of a high-powered PR campaign and a rather deceptive one at that . . .
>
> "Mrs. Lasker's opinions on research policy do not always coincide with those of many research scientists or even top NIH (National Institutes of Health) officials, but when they don't, it is often Mrs. Lasker's that prevail . . .
>
> "She arranged to have a Senate panel appointed to study cancer. . . . Most of the panel members, it turned out, were past or present members of the American Cancer Society board."[41]

During the decade of the 1970s, Mary Lasker and the American Cancer Society, in combination with the large drug companies and key cancer hospitals such as Memorial Sloan-Kettering in New York, were in virtual charge of the national cancer program. Congressmen might complain, but they could do nothing. Researchers might make discoveries which offered promise, but if the powerful business interests behind the American Cancer Society didn't approve, the researchers soon learned who was boss.

Maryann Napol's 1982 book, *Health Facts,* reported:

> "According to Washington-based observers of the medical politics scene, the NCI has both the money and the prestige within the scientific community, and the ACS has the political clout.
>
> "The American Cancer Society's political clout is exercised via the extremely influential ACS board members—some of the country's leading philanthropists, bankers and corporate executives—who also sit on key committees at the NCI. The ACS is the largest private philanthropic institution in the United States."[42]

Ralph Moss, former Assistant Director of Public Affairs at

43

Memorial Sloan-Kettering Cancer Center in New York offered these insights in his 1980 book, *The Cancer Syndrome:*

"'An ACS-controlled clique . . . dominates NCI policy and funding decisions,' according to journalist Ruth Rosenbaum. . . . 'They've (ACS) turned it into a dollar pump,' a House Appropriations committeeman added graphically.

"The days are gone when a cancer specialist would think of opposing the leadership of his field by businessmen, bankers and advertising men. The Society (ACS) now has tens of millions of dollars to distribute to those who favor its growing power, and many powerful connections to disconcert those who oppose it.

"In conclusion: the National Cancer Institute is a massively funded government bureaucracy, staffed mainly with career civil servants. Not only has its current size and structure largely been determined by outside forces, but the American Cancer Society, Memorial Sloan-Kettering, and the largest drug companies appear to exercise an important influence on the Institute's direction."[43]

Shortly after the "war on cancer" began in December 1971, the American Cancer Society decided that screening women for breast cancer was a great idea. The ACS slogan, "control cancer with a checkup and a check" (to the American Cancer Society) showed how the PR specialists at the ACS used political influence at the National Cancer Institute to initiate programs which served the ACS's financial interest. The director of the National Cancer Institute at that time, Dr. Frank Rauscher, Jr., agreed to use public funds for the project. No one bothered to consider whether women under 50 years of age really needed the exams, and whether the X-rays might cause cancer.

From 1973 to 1978, the Breast Cancer Detection Demonstration Project spent $54.6 million on screening women for breast cancer. The National Cancer Institute provided more than $46 million of the total cost. Ralph Nader's consumer watchdog group later tested a large number of the X-ray machines and found that 55% emitted more than the safe dosages. And Dr. Karl Z. Morgan, director of health physics at the Atomic Energy Commission's Oak Ridge National Laboratory, came forth to warn that diagnostic X-rays were causing cancer. The FDA hastily changed the standards within months of Morgan's 1974 warning but the NCI-ACS breast screening program went merrily forward.[23]

In an article published in the September 23, 1976 *New England Journal of Medicine,* Dan Greenberg described how the American Cancer Society pushed its program through the National Cancer Institute even though top scientists were opposed. One director of the NCI admitted, "both the American Cancer Society and the National Cancer Institute will gain a great deal of favorable publicity because they are bringing research findings to the public. . . . This will assist in obtaining more research funds."[44]

Meanwhile, some NCI officials as well as outside scientists saw very dangerous policies being promoted for the sake of the ACS's fund-raising goals. NCI's Kenneth B. Olson admitted in one memo, "This project has limited objectives and they have been pretty much dictated by the American Cancer Society." On July 16, 1973, professor Marvin Zelen at the State University of New York, Buffalo, wrote to NCI Director Rauscher that "the project is ill-conceived and is not likely to result in significant patient benefit." Then professor Malcolm C. Pike at the University of Southern California School of Medicine wrote to the NCI in December 1974 that a number of specialists had concluded that "giving a woman under age 50 a mammogram on a routine basis is close to unethical."

It took NCI a year and a half before it responded to professor Pike and announced termination of routine mammograms for women under 50. That decision was made only after John Bailar of NCI "went on a one-man speaking campaign around the country and published a serious critique of the program."[44]

NCI announced the new guideline in August 1976, but in May 1977 had to come forth with more rigid rules. Why? 75% of the women in the project were still having their annual checkups. The physicians and ACS officials simply were passing the new information to the waste basket and not telling the women!

In 1976, NCI director Frank Rauscher Jr. found a new, higher-paying job—at the American Cancer Society. Forty-six million dollars of the taxpayer's money had been used to promote a potentially dangerous test that made radiologists wealthy and provided untold free support for the American Cancer Society's own money-raising crusade. When Rauscher arrived at the ACS, he must have been received like J. P. Morgan returning from a conquest. Only the American taxpayer and the average American woman were the victims.

A year after Rauscher's departure as head of NCI, a Congressional investigation discovered that Rauscher had been charging both the ACS and NCI for trips he and his wife had made to New York and to Montego Bay, Jamaica. He should have been prosecuted but of course was not. He continued as the respected "director of research" for the American Cancer Society.

In 1978, Irwin J. D. Bross, Director of Biostatistics at Roswell Park Memorial Institute for Cancer Research commented about the cancer screening program:

> "The women should have been given the information about the hazards of radiation at the same time they were given the sales talk for mammography. . . . Doctors were gung-ho to use it on a large scale. They went right ahead and X-rayed not just a few women but a quarter of a million women. . . . A jump to the exposure of a quarter of a million persons to something which could do them more harm than good was criminal—and it was supported by money from the federal government and the American Cancer Society." (Quoted in H. L. Newbold, *Vitamin C Against Cancer,* 1979.)

One woman who was cured of breast cancer through a nutritional approach reported her experience with mammography as follows:

> "In six months my lumps in my breast were gone. . . . I had not had surgery. . . . I did not tell anyone (outside my family) I had cancer. I guess I wanted to be sure myself I could do it before I would tell anyone you could lick cancer with proper lifestyle and nutrition.
>
> "Three years later in March. . . . They X-rayed my chest and found nothing. . . . In July after the X-rays, I noticed lumps in my breast again. I had just read an article in the paper that they were finding 'hard evidence that X-ray is actually causing cancers'. . . . When I discovered the lumps back again, I immediately went back on my original schedule and

diet and within 6 months again my lumps were gone. My advice to others would be—don't get X-rays taken. The radiation is too dangerous." (Quoted in Fred Rohe, *Metabolic Ecology,* footnote 129.)

Ten years after NCI's more rigid rules regarding breast exams, and despite overwhelming evidence that the breast screening program for "early" detection was worthless, the American Cancer Society refused to give up its big lie. On March 15, 1987, the ACS officially announced, "Caught early enough, breast cancer has cure rates approaching 100 percent."

Scientists knew otherwise. The February 2, 1979 issue of the *Journal of the American Medical Association (JAMA)* carried an article by Maurice S. Fox, Ph.D. of MIT. He stated, "Many women currently treated for breast cancer appear to die at a rate similar to that of the untreated . . . patients in the 19th and early 20th century. . . . No evidence of the presumed benefit of . . . early detection is apparent in terms of breast cancer mortality, even ten years later."[45]

On August 10, 1985, Peter Skrabanek of the Department of Community Health, Trinity College, University of Dublin, Ireland, produced one of the most devastating arguments against the ACS's "early detection" and mammography program (at least as it relates to orthodox treatment—surgery, chemotherapy and radiation). The article appeared in the highly regarded British medical magazine, *The Lancet:*

"The evidence that breast cancer is incurable is overwhelming. The philosophy of breast cancer screening is based on wishful thinking that early cancer is curable cancer, though no-one knows what is 'early.'

"If breast cancer is incurable, as many surgeons believe, then screening only adds years of anxiety and fear.

"Survival rates are little affected by any of the current methods used, whether it be radical or simple mastectomy, with or without radiation, and with or without chemotherapy.

"There is no evidence that early mastectomy affects survival. If the patient knew this, they would most likely refuse surgery."[46]

Skrabanek's analysis had no effect on the ACS's breast screening program or the public relations lie that "early detection" had cure rates approaching 100%. Of course, according to the ACS, a person was "cured" if they lived 5 years from the time cancer was diagnosed, so it was easy to see that "early detection" increased the "cure" rate. Tortuous definitions to arrive at tortuous truths which wouldn't stand up to common sense analysis meant that a lot of money could keep flowing to the ACS public relations specialists. But for Dean Burk of the National Cancer Institute, who had watched the ACS game for decades, it was an old story. "They lie like scoundrels," he told journalist Peter Barry Chowka.[37]

But the breast cancer screening program wasn't the only major manipulation of the U.S. government's cancer program by the ACS. Another example of how Mary Lasker exerted her will should demonstrate how perverted the national program became because of her and the ACS's unrestrained power. Not only did they have a disastrous effect on desperate and dying cancer patients, but they squandered huge public funds to promote their pet projects.

Recall how Mathilde Krim, Mary Lasker's biologist friend at Memorial Sloan-Kettering, became so impressed with interferon during her work for the Senate committee in 1970. After the "war on cancer" report was completed, Mathilde Krim went back to New York City's Memorial Sloan-Kettering and convinced officials there that they needed an interferon laboratory. Who would head it? Mathilde Krim!

After several years, Krim's enthusiasm for interferon and Lasker's political will combined to produce the third big raid on the U.S. Treasury. Another PR campaign was mounted. This time the purpose was to force the National Cancer Institute to purchase huge amounts of synthetic interferon, even though the officials didn't want it because the test results were questionable. No matter.

Edward Shorter, Ph.D., of the University of Toronto, related what happened in his book, *The Health Century*. He quotes Stephen Canter of NCI and Dr. DeVita, Director of NCI:

> Canter: "The pressure was unbelievable. Interferon was the worst example I ever saw of politicizing the scientific decision-making process."
> DeVita: "Mary pulled out every stop."

In 1979, NCI bought $9 million of interferon. It was money that could have financed dozens of alternative cancer therapies in qualified clinics across the country.

Shorter quotes Stephen Cohen at Bristol-Myers as to the result:

> "Interferon is clearly a failure. It's damn expensive and its damn toxic. So how long is a doctor going to give something to a patient that makes him feel absolutely terrible, costs a fortune, and doesn't work?"[47]

Meanwhile, the ACS continued using its power and influence to thwart cancer therapies which had produced startling clinical results. Dr. Stanislaw Burzynski of Houston had found that harmless urinary peptides were useful as a cancer treatment. The ACS put Burzynski on its *Unproven Methods List* (?!) in 1983 even though ACS admitted that Burzynski's 1977 clinical study produced improvement in 86% of patients with advanced cancer. Within 3 months, the FDA filed suit against Burzynski to stop all research. In 1985, they raided his institute and seized his records. Robert Houston's *Repression and Reform in the Evaluation of Alternative Cancer Therapies* described the man whom the ACS was identifying as a quack:

> "In August 1986, Dr. Burzynski was a featured speaker at the 14th International Cancer Congress, the most prestigious congregation in cancer research. His paper to the assembled luminaries gave the five-year follow-up results in a clinical trial of antineoplaston therapy in patients with advanced cancer: 60% of the patients obtained objective remission, 47% of the patients experienced complete remission, and 20% survived over 5 years without cancer."[48]

Medical journalist Gary Null described Dr. Burzynski's method of supplying the cancer patient with the missing peptides and the results:

> "Dr. Burzynski has treated about 1,400 patients with advanced cancer with impressive success since 1977 . . . a therapy based not on the abuse of the body's built-in defense systems but rather on the transformation of cancerous cells into healthy, normal tissue . . .
> "The body virtually heals itself . . .
> "When applied to tissue cultures, the peptides missing from

49

cancer patients actually suppressed the growth of human cancer cells . . .

"Most patients experience virtually no side effects . . .
"The Burzynski clinic in Southwest Houston operates on an outpatient basis, with the average period of care ranging from 6 months to 3 years . . .

"While he has had little success with cancer of the testicles and childhood leukemia, he has had astounding results with brain tumors, malignant lymphomas, and cancer of the bladder."[49]

The *Unproven Methods List* of the ACS is the society's way of identifying its enemies to those who support the ACS way. Helping or associating with someone on the list can end a researcher's career.

As Robert Houston recognized:

"The Unproven Methods list of the American Cancer Society, which stigmatizes alternative treatments as 'cancer quackery' and advocates 5-year jail terms for the discoverers (ACS 1982) appears to qualify in every social and legal sense as a blacklist in cancer research."[48]

Yet the Director of the ACS's *Unproven Methods List* admitted to investigative journalist Gary Null that they didn't have "the facilities or the staff" to keep up with scientific journals and correct errors concerning those whom the ACS had labeled as "quacks."[34]

The outstanding fact is that the ACS's *Unproven Methods List* is used as a major blacklist in the scientific world. The ACS spends more than 70-75% of its funds on non-research activities (administration, fund-raising, etc.) The majority of its "research" money goes to people affiliated with its board members. And yet, despite its huge financial resources, the ACS can't manage to maintain its quack list according to any scientific standards. In truth, the evidence is overwhelming that the ACS has no interest in any objective standards. The quack list is really nothing but a political hit list used against opponents of the ACS. Besides, ACS doesn't have any qualified researchers to make such assessments in any event, according to Pat McGrady who was science editor of the ACS for 25 years. He blurted out the dirty little secret to investigative journalist Peter Chowka:

50

"The ACS slogan, control cancer with a checkup and a check . . . it's phony, because we are not controlling cancer. That slogan is the extent of the ACS scientific, medical and clinical savvy. Nobody in the science and medical departments there is capable of doing real science. They are wonderful professionals who know how to raise money. They don't know how to prevent cancer or cure patients; instead, they close the door to innovative ideas. ACS money goes to scientists who put on the best show to get grants or who have friends on the grant-giving panels."[37]

For many years, the AMA's Committee on Quackery and the ACS's Committee on Unproven Cancer Management coordinated their attacks on "outsiders." As journalist Ruth Rosenbaum concluded after examining the two committees, they "form a network of vigilantes prepared to pounce on anyone who promotes a cancer therapy that runs against their substantial prejudices and profits."[5]

The American Cancer Society gets funds from the United Way. Citizens who give to the United Way or have contributions deducted from their paychecks have little idea that the ACS is a self-perpetuating business whose interference with genuinely useful cancer therapies is massive. Citizens are also not aware that the ACS does not meet the standards of the National Information Bureau, the charity watchdog. How could they? Most of their money goes into salaries, public relations campaigns, publications which attack legitimate if unorthodox therapies, and lobbying federal officials in Washington. The ACS has a staff of 3,000 people. It has 58 divisions and 3,000 local units. Its budget throughout the 1970s was over $100 million a year. During the 1980s, it was over $200 million a year. In 1985 alone, the ACS plucked $243 million from beguiled citizens who thought they were helping a worthy cause. Pat McGrady Jr. stated in 1988 that their annual windfall receipts now exceed $400 million![26]

Only a fraction of that amount goes to research. McGrady's recommendation? "Abolish the ACS. . . . That institution is a disgrace."[50]

Peter Barry Chowka's 1978 investigation of the American Cancer Society turned up the following:

"Since 1918, the National Information Bureau (NIB) has

been the recognized independent overseer of charities and other non-profit organizations. After auditing ACS in 1976-77, NIB concluded, 'Questions arise with respect to ACS' accumulation of assets beyond the amount required for its next year's budget . . . ACS has repeatedly claimed over the past several years . . . that it would have made more research grants had sufficient funds been available, a statement not substantiated by the facts of its financial position.' In other words, ACS is hoarding and investing for profit many millions of dollars contributed by the public to fight cancer, while the society claims that vital research is going begging for funds. . . . Of the money ACS spends to 'fight cancer,' 61 percent goes for staff salaries, executive travel, office supplies and other expenses; less than 5 percent is allocated to assisting patients."[37]

During the 1970s period, the ACS collected more than $1 billion from the American public. At one point, the California branch of the ACS had accumulated over $8 million which was collecting interest in California banks. At another point, the national ACS had over $200 million invested in New York banks. Its emergency fund for hot research projects was a "big" $5 million! Yet every year the drum is rolled out and two and a half million volunteers go forth to beg for more money for the Lasker relief charity. The spectacle is sickening.

Pat McGrady Jr. reminds us:

"The American Cancer Society collects around $400 million a year. . . . I have yet to see a single breakthrough that has resulted from this colossal collection of money. Surely the answer is that they have misspent it."[26]

The tiniest percentage of all that money would fund dozens of clinics, allowing them to conduct trials of cancer therapies which actually show promise or already have been proved successful. The American Cancer Society is not interested in a cure. It would go out of business. The following example should demonstrate the point:

"On April 17, 1952, the Dickinson County, Iowa chapter of the ACS ran a full page ad in the local paper, 'The Spirit Lake Beacon,' asking the society to enter the new field of investigating cancer cure claims. They cited 4 such 'cures.' The chapter was expelled from the ACS. Its chairman, Mrs.

Roy Tatman, felt compelled to declare: 'We are at a loss to know what crime we committed. We were asked to help conquer cancer. We have tried to do just that. Has the Society another motive?"[51]

David Rorvik suggested the unspoken motive in an article which appeared in the June 1976 issue of *Harper*'s:

> "The American Cancer Society, designated by charter as an 'emergency' organization which must disband the day a cure is found, has enjoyed its emergency status since 1913 and, by every indication, is determined to be its beneficiary still in the year 2013."[3]

At a minimum, the American Cancer Society, given its history since the mid-1940s when the Laskers and Elmer Bobst (a close associate of Morris Fishbein) took over, should be investigated by the U.S. Justice Department for fraud, false advertising, conspiracy and a variety of other anti-trust, monopolistic crimes. When government officials find the nerve to initiate such an undertaking and the remnants of a free press unleash their young tigers, the public may start to wake up to how it was conned out of billions of dollars to support an organization actively involved in suppressing various cures for cancer.

In this author's opinion, millions of Americans died because of what Mary Lasker and her friends did in a grand public swindle.

And the swindle continues to the present day. In September 1990, Dr. James T. Bennett of George Mason University, located in Virginia across the Potomac River from Washington, D.C., published an essay which appeared in a number of newspapers. The essay was based on a study of health research "charities" for a Washington research center. Dr. Bennett declared:

> "The American Cancer Society . . . had a fund balance of $426.2 million in 1988, and it held net investments (after depreciation) in land, buildings and equipment of $69 million. That same year, the ACS spent only $89.2 million, or 26 percent of its budget on medical research."

It isn't just the fact that the ACS is a corrupt charity deceiving the American public and needs to be exposed as a racket.

53

The real issue is that the ACS controls or influences the government's National Cancer Institute to such an extent that innovative cancer research which might put the American Cancer Society out of business is thwarted by ACS policies and back-door pressure. As Ruth Rosenbaum's 1977 exposé made evident, the ACS is a danger to the *public* interest:

> "Mention 'National Cancer Institute' to most people, even in Bethesda, Maryland (NCI headquarters), and you'll probably be 'corrected': 'You mean the American Cancer Society.'
>
> "ACS power and affluence depends on its being recognized as the sole dispenser of cancer information . . .
>
> "Why would an NCI Division Director . . . insist that his staff consult first with ACS? An NCI source . . . explains, 'If you make waves, someone will get in touch with someone else and before you know it Mary Lasker says to the NCI Director: 'We don't like your director of such and such, so maybe you should think about getting a new one.'"[5]

Someday this terrible crime is going to be spread across newspaper front pages and television screens when the current media crowd of hacks and cowards are replaced by a new generation of courageous and patriotic journalists. And then the American public is going to explode in outrage when the enormity of the American Cancer Society's crime is comprehended. And then the politicians will "suddenly" discover the issue and Congressional investigations will begin. And then the Justice Department lawyers will "suddenly" recognize the magnitude of the criminal conspiracy. And then the doctors, "scientists," power brokers and public relations specialists associated with the American Cancer Society will proclaim their ignorance and "good intentions."

Let us hope the American people insist that justice be done and that the political leaders recognize that history will judge them very severely if they sell out and try to sweep this national tragedy and monstrous wrong under the rug.

Chapter Five
# The NCI

*"For we wrestle not against flesh and blood, but against principalities, against powers, against the rulers of the darkness of this world, against spiritual wickedness in high places."*

Ephesians 6:12

The National Cancer Institute was established by Congres in 1937. Its assignment was to develop scientific research and procedures which would cure or limit cancer. Fifty years later, after billions of dollars spent on scientific egos, expensive technology and armies of bureaucrats, there is little to show for it. NCI, as described earlier, is a virtual prisoner of large drug companies, public relations organizations, and an "old boy" network of "big league scientists" who have ignored successful cancer therapies in order to pursue their institutional priorities. No quick mechanism exists to test what physicians on the front lines discover useful. Instead, elaborate laboratory notions are slowly passed down to the hospital wards for testing. Only highly organized experiments by men and women with extensive academic backgrounds, experienced in grant writing and political maneuvering, are sanctioned. The entire historical process of medical discovery has been turned on its head. As Dr. Raymond Keith Brown explained:

"With few exceptions, major advances in traditional medicine have come from basic observation of the patient and his disease and from the reasoning of individual physicians, not from the direction and consensus of committees or authority. . . . Medical scientism ignores the empirical approaches of traditional medicine. It discounts clinical observation as being 'anecdotal' and enshrines as the sole basis for valid

55

medical judgment, statistical analysis, double blind studies and the prevailing consensus of opinion."[25]

In 1988, the Toronto newspaper, *The Globe and Mail,* published a summary on the U.S. and Canadian cancer situation. The large headline read "Getting Nowhere." Among its conclusions:

"Greater percentages of people are getting cancer and dying from it each year.

"Cancer deaths have risen steadily in the past 30 years, climbing 4 to 5 per cent annually since 1960.

"Few inroads are being made in curing the most common forms of cancer, which includes most malignant tumors of the lung and many arising in the breast, colon, pancreas and skin."[11]

Through the years, National Cancer Institute officials and political leaders have failed to recognize *the primary fact* that with thousands dying every week, it is morally indefensible to pursue its scientific agenda while ignoring and opposing a variety of treatments developed by doctors or alternative practitioners which have proven successful. Why the alternative approaches work is not the issue, not for now. *That* they work should be the spur and the driving directive of the NCI. It is not.

There should be the greatest encourgement of alternative methods. An openness to "crazy approaches" that work should characterize the operations and be the stated policy of NCI. NCI should be a clearing house and protector of the innovators. Instead, NCI is the opposite, an oppressive guardian of the status quo—chemotherapy, radiation and surgery.

The prevailing attitude of the NCI and its contempt for the average citizen's right to alternative treatment was exemplified in the late 1970s by Dr. Bayard H. Morrison III, Assistant Director of NCI. He was the person in charge of evaluating alternative treatments. In a letter to the Washington Star newspaper, Dr. Morrison dismissed any cancer treatment except for surgery, radiation and chemotherapy. He either was incompetent to judge the historical effect of the three approved modalities, or was openly lying. Dr. Morrison wrote:

"For a number of years at the National Cancer Institute, I

have had the formal responsibility of dealing with problems relating to the advocacy and use of unproven methods of cancer treatment. . . . In truth, the effective cancer treatments—surgery, x-ray and chemotherapy—are often attended by unpleasant side effects. Yet all of the advances made in cancer treatment—abundantly documented in the medical literature—are due to the use of these modalities. . . . The cancer patient should have freedom of choice—not to be gulled by the pitchman, but rather to seek out the best qualified physician or physicians and to obtain more than one opinion. . . . This will constitute the basis for informed consent."[52]

I have personally interviewed alternative practitioners who had a compound which had cured lung cancer. Government officials came in and confiscated it. I have personally interviewed a woman with a terminal, inoperable brain tumor who was cured by one of the many "underground" practitioners. She has the CATscans, before and after, to prove it. The treatment took only 3 months from "terminal and inoperative" to "totally cured.". Whether the method would work on all brain tumors is irrelevant. Whether the methodology could be taught to countless physicians and even non-physician technicians is unknown. But NCI, ignoring its original mandate, has created no mechanism to deal with these novel approaches and hard, CATscan-documented realities.

For years, Dr. Herbert Shelton of Texas ran a successful clinic where he put patients with cancer and other degenerative diseases on an extended fast—no food, only liquids. Shelton oversaw 30,000 patient fasts! His method would not be the choice of the majority of cancer patients, but certainly some significant percentage of the desperate and dying would elect to try it. Shelton's record of recovery, despite the extreme method and the late stage of many of his patients' cancers, was exceptionally high. While he is now deceased, physicians who worked with him are still alive. Every cancer hospital and clinic could offer it, with physicians trained to assist in the difficult process where the body's own regenerative energies are used.

It has been reported that AIDS might be treated similarly. While the approach is risky and certainly requires physician supervision, it ought to be objectively investigated. Readers interested in one purported success should read *Roger's Recovery From AIDS*.[53]

But the case against NCI goes far beyond its failure to provide a national testing facility for the treatment of cancer. It goes far beyond NCI's reluctance to examine fairly the unorthodox therapies which have been successful. This body has ignored scientific information critical to curing cancer. It has actively participated in conspiratorial designs against physicians and qualified researchers who pursued unorthodox approaches. And it has dismissed, hidden and remained silent about presented evidence which revealed that sanctioned and economically lucrative treatments such as radiation were deadly to the patient. NCI, like the FDA, AMA and ACS, has committed crimes against the people of the United States and other nations affected by its policies and by its subterranean activities.

In 1988, a fellow of the Royal Statistical Society in London described how NCI falsified the results of a 1973 trial involving laetrile. The details are provided in Appendix E. The expert declared:

"The NCI conclusions were a total distortion of science. The underdosed and the overdosed mice were combined with those mice receiving the optimum dosage. The trial was absolutely, absurdly dishonest. The U.S. taxpayers have a right to demand their money back. NCI is an absolutely corrupt, inept, incompetent organization distorting the truth in order to support their own image and own budget."

Ben Fitzgerald's Congressional investigation in 1953 produced evidence that NCI actively hindered, suppressed and restricted the Hoxsey therapy (see chapter three). According to Judith Glassman's *The Cancer Survivors* (1983), "One NCI official admitted that the NCI had not verified any of Hoxsey's cases with the original physicians because it had been ordered not to by the National Advisory Cancer Council."[54]

Fitzgerald's 1953 Senate report also noted that he had personally examined the records of 530 cases which indicated Krebiozen was effective. It took NCI seven years to offer to do a clinical trial. When Dr. Andrew Ivy, a renowned cancer authority and leading advocate of Krebiozen, responded with terms for his participation—exceedingly reasonable terms given the intrigue and conspiracy operating against him—NCI refused to conduct the trial. Five years later, the FDA's massive multimillion dollar criminal action against Dr. Ivy and others took place. A fair, conclusive clinical trial would have been a lot easier, a lot cheaper and certainly in the public interest.

Regarding the public interest, the entire question of radiation is another area where NCI's record is disturbing. While this subject is addressed in more detail in chapter seven, the early work of Japanese researcher Kuchio Hasumi, M.D. deserves mention, particularly since NCI had the opportunity years ago to curtail radiation before it became the current multimillion dollar industry.

Dr. Hasumi's 1980 book, *Cancer Has Been Conquered,* argued that radiation not only didn't arrest cancer but actually made a cure nearly impossible:

> "Viruses cannot be killed by drugs or radiation. On the contrary, they actually become stronger. . . . Cancer cannot be cured by any form of operation. The more a surgeon cuts out, the greater the area of weakened resistance created, and as a result the cancer viruses wreak even more havoc. . . . When the cancer cells are burnt with radiation, the patient tends to improve for about one month, because the cancer cells have been temporarily destroyed. The viruses, however, have not. When the cells start to die the viruses come crawling out in order to ensure the survival of the progeny. . . . The second carcinoma will have developed resistance to it and it will not succumb to radiation again. At the end of 3 months the viruses will be reproducing rapidly, thriving on radiation, and when this happens no treatment will help . . . radiation also kills the sources of immunity."[55]

Hasumi had demonstrated the cancer "virus" at NCI in 1954!

Thomas J. Glover had isolated the cause of cancer in the early 1920s! It was a bacteria that could be filtered to the size of a virus. Even today, 65 years later, the orthodox scientists refuse to admit that bacteria have phases which can produce microbes as small as viruses. A number of independent researchers have verified this fact, but the cancer hierarchy has good reasons for denying it—continuing, massive financial gain from research and orthodox treatment. The millions of victims are not the priority.

Glover's serum was described in newspaper accounts as early as 1924. Ten cases of cancer patients cured by the serum were reported in the *Irish Journal of Cancer* in 1926! Working with his laboratory assistant Tom Deaken (the true genius) and Dr. Michael J. Scott, Glover allowed his discovery to be investigated by the Hygienic Lab, forerunner to the National Institutes of Health and the National Cancer Institute, from 1929 to 1938. They tested 35 malignant tissues and found the Glover cancer microbe in 100% of them. They refused to publish the results.

Glover twice published the results—*Studies in Malignancy* (1938) and *The Treatment of Cancer* (1940). Three hundred and twenty nine (329) cancer patients were successfully treated between 1923 and 1939.

In the early 1930s, Royal Rife successfully isolated and destroyed the cancer microbe, curing 100% of the "terminal" cancer patients in his first clinic in 1934. Newspapers reported his work in 1938. As with Glover and Deaken, Rife discovered that the cancer microbe was a bacteria which could be filtered to a viral size.

In the middle 1930s, Dr. W. M. Crofton of Ireland also identified the same or a similar microbe as the cause of cancer. Three independent researchers all discovered the same *bacteria* as the cause of cancer, and yet by 1988 the NCI still hadn't funded and has refused to examine the work. What does that tell you?

Dr. Robert E. Netterberg and Robert T. Taylor described Deaken's and Glover's 1920s findings as follows in their 1981 book *The Cancer Conspiracy:*

> "Deaken had discovered a special culture medium for isolating and growing certain bacterial microbes from cancer tissue, blood, or urine from cancer patients or animals . . .
>
> "Deaken described its unusual life cycle and its change of form, including one filterable form comparable to a virus."[56]

Dr. Crofton reported in *The True Nature of Viruses* in 1936:

> "In cancer, the fertilization of the cell-nucleus is provided

by the virus phase of the microbe. . . . The virus has the same effect on the nucleus it invades as the head of a spermatozoan, changing the nature of the cell from a peaceful citizen contributing to the welfare of the community into one whose ferments enable it to prey on its fellows."[57]

Chemotherapy does not kill viruses. Only vaccines or bio-electronic therapy work on them. Yet in the late 1980s, NCI Director DeVita recommended that all women with breast cancer be treated with both surgery and chemotherapy. In August 1988, it was announced that DeVita was leaving NCI to take a $400,000 annual compensation at Memorial Sloan-Kettering Cancer Center in New York as physician-in-chief of the cancer treatment area. And, as the Toronto *Globe and Mail* reported on June 11, 1988:

> "The upshot for patients is that (chemotherapy) treatment is becoming much more demanding. 'Brutal would be a good way to describe it,' said Dr. Gary Spitzer, a cancer specialist and professor of medicine at the University of Texas M.D. Anderson Cancer Centre in Houston."[11]

If NCI had done its job, examined and supported alternative approaches, balanced the scientific understanding against the empirical approaches of physicians, and dared oppose the financial interests of surgeons, chemotherapists and radiologists, today's mounting cancer death tolls might never have existed.

Instead, NCI created a bureaucratic haven for scientism, filled with committee procedures, payoffs, collusion with drug companies and interminable roadblocks for the truly innovative cancer fighters. Because of NCI's failure and criminal negligence, more Americans die each year than all the Americans who died in combat in World War II.

Investigative reporter Gary Null described the NCI inner workings as follows:

> "Although it may have been formed with the best of intentions, it seems that the system of peer review breeds corruption; people who have political clout can get what they want. If the NCI wants a grant approved, it puts people on the peer review board who will approve it. One doctor described a peer review board as an old boys club. The 'boys' sit around and hand out money to each other."[34]

One such "boy" was Dr. Phillippe Shukik of the Eppley Institute in Nebraska. Dr. Shukik was a member of the National Cancer Advisory Panel as well as a paid representative to the NCI for several of the largest corporations in America. During the decade of the 1970s, Dr. Shukik's Eppley Institute received $26 million from NCI. It produced nothing noteworthy and NCI finally was publicly criticized by the Comptroller General for the waste (how about fraud?).[56]

Ralph Moss, former Assistant Director of Public Affairs for Memorial Sloan-Kettering Cancer Centre in New York described the practical outcome of such incestuous grant/peer review relations:

"A new grant request must therefore be approved by a wide variety of scientists, bureaucrats, and businessmen. It must be the result of a *consensus* of opinion among these many individuals. Almost by definition, however, such an appliction must be well wtihin the bounds of conventional science. These 'cumbersome constraints' make it difficult, if not impossible, for radically new ideas to be approved by the NCI."[43]

In 1978, U.S. Senator John Melcher spoke out against this "old boy" peer review system. Ten years later, nothing has changed. The paper and the committees proliferate. The number of people dying from cancer increases. Senator Melcher:

"If we are just going to be brokering out these grants on the basis of who has published a paper that passes some peer group as the only criteria, then I dare say we will be fumbling in this morass of inclusive research forever and ever."[7]

The brochures available to help researchers prepare a grant proposal would be rather amusing, if one were not aware of the "old boy networks" which make requests for funding of an innovative approach essentially a waste of time, and if the 10,000 Americans scheduled to die every week because of past NCI cover-ups and timidity could be ignored.

Then there is the issue of NCI's love of drugs and its various institutional coverups which constitute crimes against humanity. In October 1981 *The Washington Post* investigated some of the rot. Their findings included:

"A one year study by the Washington Post has documented 620 cases in which experimental drugs have been implicated in the deaths of cancer patients . . . And they amount to merely a fraction of the thousands of people who in recent years have died or suffered terribly from cancer experiments."

One FDA official was quoted as follows by the *Washington Post*:

"Sometimes there is little regard for people's lives . . . A hospital tested a new National Cancer Institute drug . . . on children. Their kidneys were lost within days. This was no big deal because new drugs are routinely given out with literally no safeguards for people."

The article continued:

"In the vast majority of drug experiments, it is not uncommon for none or 1 or 2 of *hundreds* of patients to benefit from the drug."

The article ended with this sad comment on political courage and leadership which *has not changed one iota* a decade later:

"These human experiments have gone largely unchallenged and unquestioned by Congress, the medical profession and the scientific community at large."

The decades-long misuse of drugs was caused by intense American Cancer Society support for chemotherapy and NCI *attitudes which had no scientific basis*. And this was further complicated by NCI antagonism against outsiders with innovative approaches. The case of scientist Lawrence Burton, Ph.D. is probably the most famous in recent years, and one of the most revolting in the past 50 years. The full details can be found in articles cited as footnotes 48, 49, 54 and 59.

Burton and his colleagues managed to shrink tumors in mice within *hours* and published their findings in 1962. In 1966, at an American Cancer Society conference and then again at the New York Academy of Medicine, the procedure was demonstrated to cancer specialists. Soon a leading official of the ACS purportedly offered Burton a $15,000 grant if he would reveal the secrets of the technique to NCI and Sloan-

Kettering. When Burton refused, an NCI official purportedly offered him a $500,000 grant for the rights. NCI sent Burton a letter saying the money was approved and asked him to mail them the technical details. But then, apparently through a bureaucratic slip-up, a second letter announced the grant had been rejected. It appears that it was the intention of the NCI to promise money, obtain the secrets, then withdraw the offer and copy the technique to gain credit for it.

Within a few months, all of Dr. Burton's research funding was cut off, invitations to speak stopped, and the articles he submitted for publication were rejected for the first time. He remained senior investigator and senior oncologist (tumor specialist) at St. Vincent Hospital in New York during the period 1966-1973. Then, in 1974, he established a clinic on Long Island and shortly afterward a magazine article (*New York* magazine, July 29, 1974) about his research gained the attention of the U.S. Senator from Ohio, Howard Metzenbaum. Senator Metzenbaum pressed NCI to investigate. NCI sent Dr. William Terry to Burton and once again money was purportedly offered if Burton would only reveal his technique. Burton again refused.

In 1975, Burton and his associate Frank Friedman, Ph.D. filed for 3 patents which were granted. But then the FDA refused to permit clinical trials. According to medical scholar Robert G. Houston, based on reports from the Burton patients' support group:

> "FDA kept sending pages of questions to be answered in what seemed to be a policy of foot-dragging; some of these were quite irrelevant yet would require studies of years. The 'endless questions' technique had been used to block . . . ˉother nonconventional therapies in the past."[48]

In July 1975, the Bahamas granted permission to Burton to treat cancer patients, despite efforts by NCI to stop the approval. In 1976, Burton's Bahamian clinic opened and a steady stream of Americans with cancer began flying to the Caribbean.

In 1978, Dr. William Terry of NCI flew to the Bahamas to investigate once again the man to whom Terry had purportedly offered funds in 1974. Dr. Terry's original meeting occurred because of pressure from Senator Metzenbaum. The resulting hostility between Dr. Burton and Dr. Terry obviously insured that Dr. Terry was one of the worst possible choices for objective evaluation of Burton's success in the Bahamas.

At a Congressional hearing in 1986, Dr. George Melcher, the former chairman of the Columbia College of Physicians and Surgeons, testified that he witnessed the meeting of the NCI's Dr. Terry with Burton in the Bahamas. According to Dr. Melcher, the NCI official contemptuously ignored Burton's records which documented tumor remissions. Dr. Melcher testified:

> "It soon became clear that Dr. Terry and the others, excepting Dr. Charles, had no interest in looking at the records. I was very angry as a lot of effort had gone into preparing the records properly and there were representatives of my government doing the kind of job that was to me despicable. I was interested in building a record, good or bad, that they could have based a judgment on, but there was no interest on their part . . .
>
> "I heard a short time later that a report had been released. The statements in the report were absolutely untrue because they didn't happen. There was no evaluation of the patients or of the records. I was there and you can't lie to me about something I've been a part of. I was not only shocked, I was angry. I just didn't feel like people at that level of government should behave in that manner. I don't like dishonesty, particularly in that situation. I felt it was blatantly dishonest . . .
>
> "I'd like to make the final point that the group that came in 1978 from the NCI . . . clearly had only one objective—to turn in a report to put pressure on the Bahamian Government to close the clinic. The report was dishonest and untrue and I have no problem in standing behind that. They were unsuccessful in their attempt and I'm sure that was a big disappointment to them."[58]

By 1980, Burton reported a 59% tumor regression rate after four years in Bahamas, with 16% achieving complete remissions. Independent studies by qualified medical researchers in later years revealed similar success.

Nevertheless, in July 1985, using trumped up charges from NCI, Bahamian officials closed the clinic. When the NCI evidence was exposed as "tainted" during the Congressional hearings in January 1986, Burton's clinic was allowed to reopen in March 1986. An independent clinical trial using Burton's method was finally being considered in the summer of 1988 by the Office of Technology Assessment (OTA), an agency of the United States Congress. But the OTA investigation was headed by a former vice-president of Memorial Sloan-Kettering in New York. A syndicated column by Jack Anderson as early as December 13, 1987 questioned the man's qualifications since he also owned stock in a company making chemotherapy products. By the summer of 1988, one highly respected scholar associated with the OTA assessment was stating that OTA was "not being objective." They had eliminated critical information from her report because it supported alternative cancer therapies. The final report published in 1990 was a "well-written whitewash". It was filled with deceit and ignored the real issues.

NCI remains adamantly opposed to the Burton therapy which at one time it was eager to purchase through a phony grant. According to journalists Gary Null and Leonard Steinman, "Dr. Gregory Curt, deputy director of the division of cancer treatment at the NCI, recently described Burton's serum to the press. 'The stuff is junk . . . I wouldn't give it to a dog.'"[59]

Yet experiments with dogs having advanced cancer have also shown 50% remissions. And similar serums, based on Burton's original discoveries, were being developed at Memorial Sloan-Kettering, financed by NCI grants!

Null and Steinman concluded that "it is clear that Dr. Lawrence Burton is saving more cancer patients who are terminally ill than any conventional cancer-treatment center in the United States."[59]

In his 1988 book, *Complete Guide to Healing Your Body Naturally,* Gary Null provided the following information on Burton's "IAT" treatment of cancer:

> "Immuno-Augmentative Therapy consists of injections of four blood proteins that Dr. Burton discovered and is able to isolate. These proteins are essentially responsible for the control and even shrinkage of tumors . . .

"Dr. Burton's therapy does not attempt to shrink a tumor directly or intervene in the growth of a cancer. It is designed only to 'augment an immune mechanism in the patient.' The stimulated immune mechanism itself is then responsible for attacking the tumor . . .

"The patient can produce only so much antibody and so much deblocking protein. Thus we have to *augment* these proteins—once a day, twice a day . . . as many as six to eight times a day . . .

"Dr. Kunderman, leading cancer specialist: 'I know of carcinoma of the pancreas, which in my experience was such a lethal, terrible carcinoma, with remission for as long as 8 or 9 years' (as a result of IAT Therapy)."[49]

Dr. Burton gave up on the NCI years ago. He has opened a second clinic in Germany. Another is planned for Mexico. Then perhaps China. They will be franchised like McDonald's, all self-sufficient. Americans with cancer will be denied Burton's treatment because of NCI officials such as Dr. Terry and his bogus investigations, but citizens of other countries will have the opportunity to choose Burton's therapy. The American public should be outraged.

Since its inception in 1937, NCI has failed to achieve even minimum results, has pursued institutional self-interest, and has been coerced by private organizations into blatant acts against the public interest. NCI thwarts dozens of possible cancer therapies which have been successful in small scale demonstrations. It conducts vendettas against those who are not part of its clique. It actively conspires with other federal agencies and private interests to legally harass or suppress promising alternative therapies, and it is organized to pursue erudite specialist curiosity which, while occasionally relevant, appears frequently to be both insignificant and in conflict with the public's immediate needs.

NCI spends *one and a half billion dollars a year* to ignore cancer therapies which work, to fund its old boy network, and to actively suppress researchers such as Burton. While this is happening, 10,000 Americans die of cancer every week!

Two remedies are essential: (1) a vast restructuring which includes elimination of many mediocre careerists as well as a full scale purge of corrupted senior officials; (2) the appointment of a hound dog of a director who will drive the agency into areas it has avoided and who has some kind of direct, on-going reporting obligation to the American public.

The first report should acknowledge that past NCI officials committed crimes against humanity. Unless that truth be widely known and its perpetrators named, condemned and punished, justice cannot be served and similar evils will occur in the future.

The enormity of this crime cannot be ignored. Irwin D. Bross, Ph.D., author or co-author of more than 350 publications on biostatistics, epidemiology, cancer research and public health, exposed the critical issues in *Crimes of Official Science* (1988)[148] and *Perspectives on Animal Research* Vol 1. (1989).[149] He described how incontestable statistical facts show that high doses of chemotherapy—"a key doctrine of the National Cancer Institute (NCI)"—killed patient's defense systems and not the cancer. He revealed how "widespread attitudes among cancer researchers, which I recognized during years of work within the cancer establishment" led to lucrative scientific fraud and the use of high toxicity doses of drugs that clearly destroyed human immune systems, not the patient's cancer.

This is the basis of the charge of crimes against humanity. For almost 25 years, evidence has shown that officially sanctioned procedures have been killing people. Top scientists and physicians have "gone along" in order to further their careers. A form of institutionalized insanity has been at the core of the opposition to non-toxic, alternative treatments which have been kept illegal and ruthlessly squelched by defenders of the status quo. The butchers of surgery, chemotherapy and radiation have grown rich on the mutilated bodies of millions of innocent victims while public health officials sold their souls.

Chapter Six
# Energy Medicine

*"There is nothing more difficult to carry out, nor more doubtful of success, nor more dangerous to handle, than to initiate a new order of things."*

Machiavelli (1469-1527)

The cure for cancer will not come from chemotherapy, radiation, surgery or breakthroughs from within the government agencies, for reasons which have already been made clear. The cure for cancer has existed for many years. It lies in the area of "energy medicine" and the only reason desperate and dying cancer victims do not know of it and cannot obtain it is the ignorance and opposition of the orthodox medical hierarchy. When the public demands access to energy medicine as their right, then the barriers will fall as media and political forces converge and begin supporting these long-suppressed therapies.

Dr. Robert O. Becker, a pioneer in the field of energy medicine, stated in a 1987 interview:

"the concepts of energy medicine—in the sense that the energies involved are electrical or electromagnetic—are potent concepts. . . . The ability to affect things medical that we do not have the capacity to do at present is enormous. This field needs to be explored for a wide variety of reasons, not only environmental but also in relation to medical treatment, because it offers such great advantages over the present drug-chemical concept."[60]

Becker points out that it has been known since the 1800s that cancer is electrically negative. And electricity was linked to the Chinese system of acupuncture by Louis Berlioz as early as 1816. The Chinese determined thousands of years ago that:

> "there is an electrical wiring system in the body where all organs and systems have terminal points in various locations on the body, all of them being represented in the hands and feet."[61]

In 1889, the electronic genius Nikola Tesla described his research relating electromagnetic waves to the cells of living organisms. He announced his findings to the American Electro-Therapeutic Association. In other words, electronics as therapy was widely supported as early as the late 19th century. Yet a hundred years later it is only beginning to re-emerge because of the successful political suppression brought about by the AMA, drug companies and federal agencies. A century has been lost.

In 1925, George Lakhovsky, a French scientist, published studies which showed that plants inoculated with cancer could be healed with simple radio frequencies. Lakhovsky's paper describing his studies, "Curing Cancer With Ultra Radio Frequencies," appeared in the U.S. publication, *Radio News,* in February 1925:

> "A first plant was submitted to the effect of the radiation one month after being inoculated with cancer; at this time small tumors of the size of a cherry were visible upon it. This plant was submitted to the rays twice, for three hours each time. During the following days, the tumors continued to grow rapidly in the same way as those on plants which had not been submitted to the effect of radiations. However, 16 days after the first treatment, the tumors began to shrink and dry up. A few days later the tumors were entirely dried up and could be very easily detached from the limb of the plant by merely touching them. The drying action of the radio frequency radiation is selective and affects only the sick part of the plant. Even the inside sick tissues were destroyed, although they were next to healthy cells in the center of the limb, showing that the radiations had not affected the healthy parts.
>
> "Another plant was treated in the same way, except that it was exposed 11 times, for 3 hours each time to the radiations of the oscillator. Sixteen days after the first exposure the

tumors, which were rather large as shown in one of the photographs, began to shrink and dry up and were easily detached from the limb exactly as in the first case. Again in this case the healthy parts of the plant were not affected in the least. A third plant exposed to the radiation for nine hours each, was cured in the same manner as the two others. Sixteen plants also inoculated with cancer, were left without treatment. They have tumors in full activity, several of which are very large. These experiments show conclusively that plants inoculated with cancer can be treated and cured by means of the ultra radio frequency vibrations whereas surgical treatment fails.

"Such are the results of my researches with plants. At the present time similar experiments are being carried out with animals and it seems that the effect on cancerous animals is the same as on cancerous plants.

"I am highly pleased to present my theory and the results of my work in a scientific review of the United States, this great country which has always been in the lead in the fight against this terrible sickness, cancer, and whose sympathy and help I would greatly appreciate."[62]

In 1926, George Lakhovsky built a device for treating human diseases. Lakhovsky was granted a U.S. patent in 1934, but it was ignored and suppressed by the medical and scientific authorities of the time. Modern Lakhovsky devices are still built by individual engineers and alternative health practitioners, but there has been little interest or formal research, and no first-rate clinical studies by the army of cancer specialists being paid billions of dollars of the public's money. The current devices are not FDA approved and all carry a statement "for experimental use only." If the NCI and FDA were fulfilling their responsibilities, NCI would have 50 years of research into Lakhovsky and FDA would have established manufacturing standards which ensured quality. Of course, that could result in millions of people curing their own early-stage cancers in their own homes, totally eliminating the physicians and drug companies.

In 1933, Dr. George Crile, a renowned surgeon, gave a prophetic speech to the American College of Surgeons. Crile made the front page of the *New York Times* as he predicted future physicians would be able to diagnose and treat patients before their diseases became apparent. The method: energy medicine. The *New York Times* for October 9, 1933 reported:

"The medical man of the future, Dr. Crile said, would 'tune in' on the living body as one does now on the ordinary radio. By 'listening in' to the short-waves and the long-waves, transmitted by the various organs, he would hear the 'symphony' played by the living organism and would determine the rhythms of the 'dance of life.'

"Long before there was any outward evidence of disease, the physician-radio-engineer of the future would thus be enabled to tell by the 'reception' of the 'life-waves' whether they were playing a melody of health or whether they were signaling an SOS."[63]

Crile's prediction is exactly what happens today in the most advanced medical healing, using sophisticated electronic instruments.

In 1934, Royal R. Rife of San Diego accomplished what may be the greatest achievement by any single individual involved in 20th century energy medicine. After years of research based on a light microscope of his own invention, which to this day has not been duplicated, he was able to destroy the virus that caused cancer using a specific radio frequency. This was done hundreds of times in laboratory studies and then in a 1934 clinic, with 16 "terminal" cancer patients. All recovered. A number of subsequent clinics in the years 1935-38 accomplished similar cancer cures using a painless, non-invasive, 3-minute treatment every third day. The AMA virtually stopped the Rife treatment in 1939, first by threatening the physicians using Rife's instrument, then by forcing Rife into court.

In 1938, the *San Diego Union* reported on Rife's historic breakthrough:

"Discovery that disease organisms, including one occurring in dread cancer, can be killed by bombarding them with radio waves tuned to a particular length for each kind of organism, was claimed today by a San Diego scientist, Royal R. Rife. . . .

"The discovery promised fulfillment of man's age-old hope for a specific destroyer of all his infectious diseases, although

Rife avoided any claim that he had established this yet. He announced his work in the conservative manner of scientists, but his reports indicated the great promise in their telling of the successful bombardment of thousands of cultures of organisms, including almost all kinds known to afflict mankind.

"Organisms from tuberculosis, cancer, sarcoma, the tumor resembling cancer but not so mortal as it; deadly streptococcus infection, typhoid fever, staphylococcus infection and two forms of leprosy were among the many which the scientist reported are killed by the waves. He said that his laboratory experiments indicated that the method could be used successfully and safely on organisms at work in living tissues.

"'We do not wish at this time,' Rife commented, 'to claim that we have 'cured' cancer, or any other disease, for that matter. But we can say that these waves, or this ray, as the frequencies might be called, have been shown to possess the power of devitalizing disease organisms, of 'killing' them, when tuned to an exact wave length, or frequency, for each different organism. This applies to the organisms both in their free state and, with certain exceptions, when they are in living tissues' . . .

"The San Diego man explained that he found that different disease organisms have particular, individual chemical constituents and this led him to suspect that the organisms were electrical in nature and character and might coordinate with variable electrical frequencies. His observations have been confirmed by certain British medical researchers, who say they found that each kind of disease organism has a distinct radio wave length."[64]

During the period 1935 to early 1939, the leading laboratory for electronic or energy medicine in the United States, located in New Jersey, was independently verifying Rife's discoveries. In late 1938, the AMA began its crackdown on physicians curing cancer and other diseases with Rife's instrument. And then in March 1939, while the director of the New Jersey laboratory, Dr. J. C. Burnett, was visiting Rife in California, his laboratory was "mysteriously" burned to the ground at 3 a.m.

The *New York Times* headline reporting the disaster read, "$250,000 Fire Razes Mystery Workshop, New Type of

Therapy Believed Goal in Huge Laboratory on Palisades Estate." The article read:

"Alpine, N.J., March 12—The mysterious laboratory that Dr. John Clawson Burnett built on his 400-acre estate here fifteen years ago was destroyed by fire today, with the probable loss of all the equipment and records of experiments that he had hoped would make the world a better place to live in. . . . The Burnetts were said to be returning at once from a visit to California, where they had planned to stay until the end of this month . . . police and fire officials set it (the damage) at a minimum of $250,000. At the time the building was constructed the cost was set at that figure, and Dr. Burnett said he was putting twice that much into 'this experiment'. . . . There are eight other buildings on the land. . . . There was not a particle of magnetic substance—not an iron nail in the building.

"At the outset Dr. Burnett named the place the Burnett-Timken Research Laboratory and said the commercial possibilities of his work did not concern him. But other than declare that he would deal entirely with electronic energy in its relationship to the human body, he disclosed nothing of his plans. . . . The fire was discovered by Motorcycle Patrolman William Ettell of the Palisades Interstate Park police at 3:30 a.m. Seventy-five men from five companies . . . were unable to check the blaze until late this afternoon. . . . Neighbors were inclined to put the damage much higher than the officials had— the figure ran as high as $3,000,000."[65]

In 1940, Arthur Yale M.D. of San Diego reported to a convention of the California State Homeopathic Medical Society the results he had achieved with Rife's instrument. His talk included the following case studies:

"With this apparatus the patient suffering from a malignant growth can be bombarded with the frequency which will destroy the . . . virus. Having used this apparatus for almost two years, the writer has had the satisfaction of witnessing the disappearance of every malignant growth, where the patient had remained under treatment, these included epitheliomas, carcinomas and some of undetermined origin . . . it appears to the writer that the credit for the disappearance of the growths should be given to the destruction of the . . . virus.

74

"For purpose of elucidating, a few of the more remarkable cases are given in detail.

"Mrs. L., age 49 years, came to me on June 5, 1939. . . . X-ray pictures showed a mass the size of a cantaloupe at pyloric end of the stomach. . . . Treatments were commenced immediately. . . . Pain rapidly disappeared and on October 20, 1939, a picture was made showing the entire mass had disappeared.

"Mrs. A., age 59 years, came to me on January 7, 1939. . . . X-ray pictures showed irregular mass at pyloric end of the stomach the size of an orange with almost completed occlusion, the lymphatic involvement extending both upwards and downwards. . . . Rife-ray . . . were given three times a week . . . pain disappeared. . . . At the end of five months the mass entirely disappeared. . .

"Mr. C., age 53 . . . three of our leading surgeons had diagnosed the case as inoperable carcinoma of the rectum. There was a large irregular shaped mass in the rectum the size of a grapefruit which had to be pushed out of the way before he could have a stool. . . . Treatments were instituted, pain disappeared before the completion of the first week's treatment. . . . The entire mass disappeared at the end of sixty days. . .

"Mrs. J., age 58. . . . The patient had lost sight in her left eye and the case was referred to Dr. Sherman, who diagnosed carcinoma of the retina. He advised immediate enucleation to save the right eye. In October 1938 I installed the Rife ray machine and discontinued all treatments except the Rife ray three times a week in this case. In December the vision returned to the eye and Dr. Sherman said the growth had entirely disappeared, leaving a scar on the retina. In January 1939, Dr. Sherman reported that all the growth had disappeared and also the scar on the retina, and the vision was the same in both eyes.

"I have quoted in detail the four cases which were far advanced, each one of which would probably have proved fatal within 90 days. . . The effect of the Rife ray on all malignant growth is so remarkable and so universally satisfactory that I felt this society should have the first report and the credit for advancing what evidently promises to be the first positive treatment for the ever-increasing curse of cancer and its resultant fatalities."[66]

75

Dr. Yale was naïvely optimistic. Rife's treatment was ruthlessly suppressed by the AMA's Morris Fishbein. Doctors were paid off to lie. Others meekly walked away from Rife. Two men who tried to promote the Rife instruments were jailed for three years in a court case where medical documentation was not permitted to be introduced as evidence.

Only in 1987, following publication of *The Cancer Cure That Worked*, did interest in Rife revive.[67]

It was because the NCI and FDA had cooperated in suppressing a number of breakthrough cancer cures that Rife and his successors weren't able to patent their discoveries, and that national standards of safety and effectiveness weren't established.

The discoveries of Tesla, Lakhovsky, Rife and other scientists were conveniently lost or ignored. The "professional" cancer investigators only began to investigate energy medicine long after the historic breakthroughs already had happened. As always, it was slow, academic-oriented and periodically interrupted by dirty politics from the vested interests of the medical establishment.

Robert O. Becker, M.D. and Andrew A. Marino, Ph.D. put forth in their 1982 book, *Electromagnetism and Life,* that "the modern concept of electrobiology can be considered to have originated" in 1941 with a famous lecture given by Albert Szent-Gyorgyi. Of course, by then Rife and the physicians working with his instrument already had cured a significant number of "terminal" cancer patients. No matter. Academic medicine has its own history and woe to those not part of the club.

Szent-Gyorgyi, 1937 Nobel Prize winner for discovering Vitamin C, delivered his groundbreaking lecture on March 21, 1941 in Budapest. Becker and Marino summarized its significance as follows:

> "It is evident that over the past 50 years a steadily increasing body of scientific knowledge has been acquired indicating the existence of functional electromagnetic properties within living organisms. Not in the mystical, vitalistic sense proposed by Galvani but resting upon modern knowledge of the electronic state of matter and electronic conducting mechanisms, as originally proposed by Szent-Gyorgyi."[68]

In 1976, Szent-Gyorgyi published *Electronic Biology and Cancer*. In it, he specifically argued that there was no conflict between his discoveries in electrobiology and the virus theory of cancer. Rife's original work and practical success in the 1930s was not in contradiction with the father of electronic medicine, as recognized by the academics. Szent-Gyorgyi wrote:

"It may be well to try to clarify here the relation of the presented material to the virus theory of cancer. As a biologist I can discuss only the biological end of the story. What is clear to me is that cell division is brought about by a very specific, involved, and subtle biological mechanism. This mechanism has been built by Nature through millions, if not billions of years. Viruses cannot produce such a mechanism. What they can do is only to disturb the regulations of this mechanism, set the machine going, not create it. They can set it in motion by creating disorder. So the virus theory and theory presented in this book are not contradictory, but complementary."[69]

What Rife had done was to electronically destroy the virus, thus removing at least one critical cause of disorder, enabling the body to re-establish order. Modern bio-electronic instruments go much further, working on the principle that each organ and system has its own optimal energy pattern that can be re-established without the damaging effects of chemotherapy, radiation and surgery. Rife's capacity to destroy the viruses which caused disease and the capacity of modern instruments to *enhance* organs and systems are not in conflict. Rather they can complement each other and accelerate recovery from cancer and other life-threatening diseases.

In the early 1950s, Dr. Reinholdt Voll of Germany developed a system to test electronically the acupuncture points of the body. Acupuncture originated as a system of medicine in China thousands of years ago and has slowly gained grudging scientific acceptance in the West during the second half of the 20th century. By 1986, Dr. Julian N. Kenyon of England could declare that there "have been many papers on the subject of acupuncture, sufficient even to satisfy the most conservative medical journals that there is convincing evidence that it works."[70]

But in the 1950s, Voll was working either alone or with

only a few qualified researchers. Voll measured the ancient points on hands and feet, and compared his readings to the known diseases of many patients. He then discovered that various medications could be tested while his electronic instrument was linked to the patient. In this way, he determined whether or not a specific medication was good or bad for a given patient. (Imagine what testing chemotherapy this way *before* the patient received it would show!)

Shortly thereafter, during the period 1955-58, another German doctor, Franz Morell, began working in the field of bio-electronics or electromagnetic oscillations. In 1958, he invented a method which verified the medication testing discovery of Dr. Voll. And then in the mid-1970s, Dr. Morell made another breakthrough. He began sending the electromagnetic oscillations of the medications directly into the patient! The patient did not have to take the medicine, only receive the electronic oscillations! The healing effect was the same or better.

Dr. Morell worked with an electronics engineer named E. Rasche. Today, the instruments they built are known as MORA therapy units. (MORA = *MO*rell + *RA*sche.) It is also known as "Therapy with the patient's own oscillations."

During the same period, Dr. F. A. Popp, a physicist in Germany, discovered critical physics principles which explained how bio-electronic medicine worked. According to Dr. Morell, Popp "proved that all living matter emanates photons. . . . He showed also that the emission of photons changes with the presence of homeopathic medicaments. . . . Photons are essentially electromagnetic oscillations. . . . Dr. Popp believes them to be probably the smallest elements of matter. Their frequencies are in the range of ultra-violet light. Their speed is that of the velocity of light. Furthermore, Dr. Popp proved that any biological process is caused by electromagnetic oscillations."

What does this mean for the average person? It means that instruments made by Morell and Rasche as well as more modern instruments of others based on similar principles can induce healing electronically, using the patient's own electromagnetic oscillations, feeding in health-inducing oscillations and reversing or antidoting disease oscillations. The therapy has been in existence now for over a decade and many difficult cases have successfully been treated. Popp, Morell and others have proved that biological diseases are preceded by electromagnetic indications. Cancer and other diseases can be diagnosed and treated before the signs of cancer are evident, and with those whose cancer is obvious, the advanced therapy of energy medicine also can restore health in many instances. When the orthodox medical world "wakes up" to what already has been proved as a practical therapy, then millions of suffering victims of the old medicine will have a chance to be restored to full health.

Morell stated:

"That the effects of electromagnetic fields and oscillations are prior to all biochemical phenomenon (has been) known only for a short time and it has not yet found entrance into the common conception of the world today. . . . All biochemical phenomena are controlled and regulated by electromagnetic oscillations."[71]

In a clinical study done at UCLA and reported in *The American Journal of Acupuncture* in 1985, there was a 98% accuracy rate in identifying and separating confirmed lung cancer patients from healthy individuals. The method used bio-electronic diagnostic instruments and the acupuncture points.[72]

When American medicine recognizes the efficacy of *treating* (not only *diagnosing*) with such instruments, the North American public will become healthier rapidly, and relatively inexpensively compared to the cost of the current medical system.

Dr. Wolfgang Ludwig, D.Sc., a German physicist, provided the following example of a MORA unit's effectiveness:

"*Metastasis of testicular tumor:* A 21-year old male patient who had been partially castrated and had a cancerous lymph node removed, with subsequent radiation therapy of the draining lymph vessels. Radiographic results: malignant lymphangioma. The patient refused chemotherapy. Four MORA basic treatments caused the metastatis to disappear (radiographic follow-up: symptom-free for several years).

"The clinical cases described in the preceding section may

seem astonishing, but they are not unique. MORA therapy has been used over a hundred thousand times during the past five years. . .

"'Therapy with the patient's own oscillations' . . . has proven to be an excellent method, especially in cases which have previously been resistant to therapy. The major advantage is that the system constantly adjusts itself to the patient's situation at any given moment, since the patient and the MORA unit form a closed system. Even in cases of unclear or difficult diagnosis the treatment is always administered at the correct frequencies, since these are generated by the patient himself."[73]

The new energy instruments utilize the Chinese acupuncture points and also homeopathic remedies. Homeopathy was developed by the German physician and chemist Samuel Hahnemann (1755-1843). It was brought to the United States in 1825 and developed into a powerful medical therapy until the AMA virtually destroyed it. In 1895, there were 14,000 homeopathic physicians in the U.S. As Dr. Julian N. Kenyon relates the history of homeopathy, it almost dominated American medicine:

"The drug industry depends crucially on a sort of mass hypnosis for the continued success of its most profitable products. This effect has spread amongst the medical profession with whom it almost certainly started. The American Medical Association began the process by teaming up with the then infant drug industry and advertising its products. Of incidental interest is the fact that one of the reasons for setting up the AMA was to stamp out homeopathy. Unbelievable enough at that time homeopathy and herbal medicine seemed set to take over and dominate the American medical scene."[70]

Homeopathy is now thriving in such diverse places as India, Pakistan, Mexico, West Germany, France, England, Argentina, Brazil, and Chile. There are even a few hundred homeopathic physicians in Soviet Russia. The British and Dutch royal families are staunch supporters of homeopathic medicine.

Dr. Hahnemann created the terms homeopathy and allopathy. Allopaths are the drug-oriented AMA-type physicians who run the North American (U.S. and Canada) medical systems and oppose any substantial patient rights which would enable seriously sick people to have the option of homeopathic medicine, energy medicine, acupuncture, etc.

British medical journalist Veronica Strang described homeopathy as follows in the Canadian health newsletter, *The Missing Link:*

> "Despite its image, which is largely the result of ignorance and prejudice, homeopathy is in fact a refined system of therapeutics which has been developed with consistency and precision for over 170 years. While some of its underlying principles can be traced back to Hippocrates and other ancient healers, it was crystallized into a formal system by Samuel Hahnemann, an 18th century practitioner in Germany.
>
> "The most common explanation offered by homeopaths is that they are dealing with energy, not chemistry. They maintain that everything on earth has a 'dynamic energy' or imprint that is entirely individual, like a genetic code. In the process of potentization it is this energy that is carried over and enhanced, and it is this energy, rather than any chemical reaction, that affects the vital force of a human being."[74]

Potentization is the process by which the chosen homeopathic medicine is diluted progressively to the point where no molecule exists. Morell used vials of specific homeopathic remedies, precisely and carefully developed over the past 170 years, in combination with electromagnetic oscillations. Instead of a patient taking the homeopathic substances orally, which is the classic method of Dr. Hahnemann, Dr. Morell sent the energy from the vials into the body electronically. Thus, a future physician will only have to purchase one set of the basic homeopathic remedies. The bottles are never opened. They can be used again and again on different patients, depending on each patient's particular disease and the most appropriate remedy.

Homeopathy, acupuncture and energy medicine represent such an enormous threat to the existing medical system of drug companies, physicians trained in chemical medicine, and the various administrative officials of the public and private institutions supporting the status quo, that any recognized breakthrough involving any aspect of the three alternative methods is met by concerted opposition. In 1988, one such breach in the wall occurred.

On June 30, 1988, the prestigious British scientific journal, *Nature,* published an article which they had taken two years and four revisions to release. Independent scientists from six laboratories in four nations—France, Canada, Israel and Italy—had found that an antibody diluted to the point where every molecule of the original substance should have been eliminated still contained "something" which produced the antibody reaction. Homeopathy was on the verge of official scientific recognition. So the authorities counterattacked.

> "We are certain that these results must be wrong, but we have been unable to prove them. We are sending a team of experts to Paris to observe the research at first hand," commented *Nature*'s deputy editor to the New York Times.[75]

The Toronto *Globe and Mail* provided its readers with an insight into the scientific stakes by hinting at the rabid opposition to homeopathy:

> "The most immediate implications of the work may be that it provides a theoretical basis for homeopathic medicine. Homeopaths have traditionally diluted and shaken their natural medicines as part of their preparations."
>
> "Western science has long maintained dilution effectively destroyed any curative power of the substance. . .
>
> "'We could be looking at a kind of phenomenon that shakes the present rules of microbiology, chemistry, physics and other sciences,' Ms. Fortner said." (Patricia Fortner is a scientist at the University of Toronto who participated in the research.)[76]

Dana Ullman, in a medical newsletter, wrote what the mainstream press couldn't write, despite its obviousness:

> "This denial of the power of microdoses is reminiscent of Galileo's efforts to encourage the clergy of his time to look through his telescope. Scientists have refused to acknowledge homeopathic medicine for the past two centuries (they have refused to look through the telescope). To make matters worse, once they finally look through the telescope, they then refuse to acknowledge what they see."[77]

After *Nature* sent in its investigative team, which included the American magician James Randi, whose own background involving fraud is not entirely clean, they reported that the orthodox scientific world could relax. (Randi's lack of integrity and his disrespect for scientific objectivity were exposed by the reputable astronomer Dennis Rawlins in the October 1981 issue of *Fate* magazine. Biologist Lyall Watson later referred to Randi as "a professional magician, a consummate liar and an addicted cheat" in his 1987 book, *Beyond Supernature*.) The *Nature* team concluded, according to *TIME* magazine, "that the weird water was only a delusion . . . based on flawed experimentation." The lead French scientist whose work was being impugned, Jacques Benveniste, a laboratory head at the French National Institute of Health and Medical Research, was furious. According to *TIME*, Benveniste "compared the probe to 'Salem witch hunts and McCarthy-like prosecutions.'"[78]

As another expert commented to this author:

> "*Nature*'s editors were literally driven so insane that they had to go out and get a magician. Either that or they had to admit all the science they knew had to be thrown out."

The comical sight of the most prestigious science journal in England bringing in a disreputable American magician to help disprove a scientific finding which the established authorities did not like would be a hilarious caricature of how "professional" science purports to operate . . . unless one were aware of the financial stakes, and the millions of desperate patients whose lives hang in the balance while these deceits are played out.

According to the *British Medical Journal*, data for 24 areas of the world monitored by the United Nations indicates 6 million new cases of cancer every year. The entire world cancer rate is certainly much higher.[79]

In the early 1970s, a group of eminent scientists gathered at a conference on bio-electronic medicine sponsored by the New York Academy of Sciences. During one panel discussion, Dr. C. A. L. Bassett declared, "To go out on a limb, I would say that in 20 years, almost as much electrotherapy as chemotherapy will be used in the medical community."[80]

The prediction may still prove to be accurate, but only if there is a crisis in the next few years or a public clamor which brings about a sudden openness to electronic or energy medicine. It has not slowly evolved into scientific respectability, as Dr. Bassett seemed to assume. The cancer conspirators and medical mafia have seen to that.

To summarize, energy medicine, based on ancient (acupuncture), carefully proven (homeopathic, Rife) and recent (Voll, Morell) discoveries, now can cure cancer and other degenerative diseases according to scientific principles. The accepted mainstream modalities of chemotherapy, surgery and radiation are incapable of successfully treating cancer, as decades of statistical evidence clearly demonstrate.

Thomas E. Jones delivered a paper at the Fourth General Assembly of the World Future Society which outlines the existing knowledge:

> "Each human being, as well as each other living system, appears to have a distinctive electro-magnetic life field interpenetrating and surrounding its body.
>
> "This field and its subdivisions can be measured accurately and repeatedly.
>
> "Certain precisely specified frequencies, amplitudes, and waveforms are regularly associated with—and seem to be causally related to—healthy, electrically balanced (homeostatic) functioning of various parts of the body and of the body as a whole.
>
> "Certain other frequencies, amplitudes, and waveforms generally accompany, or serve as early warning signals of various types and degrees of disease and degeneration that disrupt this balance.
>
> "Specific kinds of instrument-mediated, non-invasive stimulation with appropriate corrective frequencies, amplitudes, or waveforms (or corresponding ingested remedies) can frequently alleviate an incipient or established pathological condition and help to rebalance the entire organism."[81]

These concepts have all been demonstrated. A number of practitioners in Europe and North America, using these energy instruments, are mastering the healing techniques associated with them. As with surgery, chiropractic or any other healing specialty, it takes time to become proficient. That process is now underway for many, many energy medicine practitioners.

And just over the horizon may exist future breakthroughs

which even now are in the prototype stage, involving the marriage of advanced physics, computers and little-known medical therapies. One such pioneer on the frontier of energy medicine is working not only on an instrument which utilizes the acupuncture points, homeopathic principles, the discoveries of Voll, Morell, Popp and others, but also advanced physics which enable him to determine the genetic disease derived from a specific grandparent, and then, applying information and energy according to recognized principles, cleanse such genetic disabilities ticking away like time bombs.

This researcher-inventor confidently states that the human body can dissolve any tumor *if* it is given the right information and provided the right biochemistry.

It may seem far-fetched to envision a day when the genetic diseases derived from a grandparent can be not only diagnosed energetically, but eliminated before they manifest. Yet as far back as the 1930s, doctors working with terminal cancer patients were recognizing such links. Dr. Josef Issels wrote in October 1936:

> "I have learned to trace back an illness through the generations. A grandfather had stomach pains. His son had an ulcer—and now the grandson has cancer in the stomach. That cancer progressed through three generations."[82]

Yet, with all its promise, energy medicine also can be dangerous. Medically ignorant engineers and unscrupulous multi-level marketers making unsubstantiated claims for their expensive "black boxes" to desperate cancer patients could set back for decades the development of energy medicine. As energy medicine pioneer Dr. Robert Becker knowledgeably affirmed and warned in his brilliant *Crosscurrents*:

> "We are now beginning to understand how almost vanishingly small electrical currents act upon certain cells to produce healing and, in some instances, to cause cancer cells to return to normal . . .
>
> "If we can provide energy medicine with respectability at this crucial time, we can clear the way for future developments that will expand the horizons of this field beyond anything we can now conceive . . .
>
> "But our enthusiasm must be tempered with prudence . . .

This is an area we should enter with caution . . .

"There is a very real hazard of stimulating other cancer growth with . . . electricity."

Meanwhile, the proponents of today's orthodox medicine, like generals still fighting a lost war, continue planning more and more chemotherapy trials for their unwitting human guinea pigs. Like frenzied Dr. Strangeloves running wild in a dark tower, they seem to have lost all sense of balance, scientific integrity and responsibility toward the sick and the suffering.

Energy medicine waits for its time, its advocates growing in number, the history of its effectiveness and scientific verification accumulating, the number of competent practitioners increasing—all waiting for the chance to be allowed to save the desperate and the dying.

Chapter Seven
# A Vast Conspiracy

*"The Inquisition is still with us. It is called the Food and Drug Administration. It is called the National Cancer Institute. It is called the American Cancer Society and the AMA. They are allied together to destroy innovation in modern times."*

Robert G. Houston[26]

The evidence that a vast conspiracy exists to prevent the use of new discoveries and known alternative therapies in the treatment of cancer is overwhelming. That there is a determined effort by vested interests to continue using drugs, radiation and surgery, despite substantial documentation that they don't work, no longer can be dismissed. A coterie of influential institutions and people who benefit from the orthodox cancer therapies continues to subvert the laws, scientific standards and moral principles in order to keep their power, prestige and profits. Millions of people die because of these vested interests. Careers of dedicated scientists are destroyed. The media is shamefully manipulated and intimidated. And timidity and fear spread through the corridors of otherwise honorable political and scientific institutions. Fundamental principles upon which American society is based are threatened.

High officials of the AMA, FDA, NCI and ACS, along with their associates in the drug companies, lawyers, lobbyists, bankers, university chiefs and various investors, are guilty of contributing, by their actions or by their silence, to a monstrous crime against humanity. The number of innocent people who have died because of this conspiracy of greed, ignorance and power exceeds the slaughter perpetrated by Hitler or Stalin. It is not an exaggeration to state that America has had on its soil for many years a clique whose evil is comparable to the worst crimes of the totalitarian madmen.

That this conspiracy has been allowed to exist so long, despite the periodic exposure of its effects, indicates that our political and media leaders either have been corrupted, are terrified of confronting the plot, or have not been doing their jobs. In any case, it is now very late in the game. The health of the entire nation is imperiled.

There is no "quick fix." Citizens must begin in their own private ways to force change. They must talk to their neighbors, give speeches at Rotary and other community organizations, form alternative cancer societies, petition their Congressmen, and in general refuse to be silent. They must be prepared to be opposed and must consider that any serious initiatives against the monster could be personally dangerous. But just as Americans risked their lives against Nazism and other totalitarian forces, they must realize that defending freedom requires sacrifice.

From 1964 to 1974, a vast conspiracy organized by the cancer cartel and totally financed by the drug companies attacked hundreds of individuals perceived as a threat. The "Coordinating Conference on Health Information," using the FDA, postal authorities, the U.S. Public Health Service and the Federal Trade Commission, conducted raids on alternative health practitioners throughout the nation. The targets were selected by the ACS, the AMA and others. The media, like sheep, reported on the "quack crackdown." Finally, after citizen complaints reached an uproar, the conspirators pulled back, quietly secured positions in private and public agencies, and took a less conspicuous role. But the war against alternative health quietly continued. Key safety and health regulations and their enforcement are now in the hands of, or are directly influenced by, the men and women in the service of the cancer conspirators.[83]

To take one example of what these national campaigns of suppression produce, let us look at radium and the radiology treatments which should have been stopped years ago. When the critics are silenced, alternative methods stopped, new scientific discoveries censored, and public information controlled, then deadly but lucrative technologies such as radiation treatment flourish.

Radiology was originated by Dr. Emile Grubbe in 1896 but it was not until the 1930s that it began to be used to any extent. Following World War II, the government and the mass media began massive campaigns to "sell" radiation to the public. It fit nicely with the atomic energy program and therefore had a dual constituency—government officials and the growing number of radiologists who had a personal financial stake in achieving broad public acceptance.

Thus a mass propaganda effort in radiology took place in the late 1940s and 1950s. People literally became human guinea pigs, as James T. Patterson made clear in his book *The Dread Disease:*

"In 1951 *Collier's* published a lavishly illustrated article showing a woman lying, helpless and alone, in a huge vault at Brookhaven laboratories in New York. She was being 'blasted' by atoms of boron, which were 'exploding' the tumor in her brain. The writer explained that this therapy, being used for the first time and with no known results, was a 'spectacularly promising phase of atomic research.'

"Upset at the expectations aroused by such hyperbole, some critics warned that radiation therapy was at best an inexact science, at worse highly dangerous to patients."[39]

Despite such concerns, radiation therapy expanded. By the late 1960s, radiation therapy was the standard treatment following surgery for breast cancer. It was curtailed only when studies began showing it offered *no survival* advantage. By 1974, the respected British medical journal, *The Lancet,* reported that radiation following breast surgery *increased* the death rates.

"An increased mortality in early breast cancer can be correlated to the routine use of local postoperative irradiation. The decreased survival is statistically significant. Of controlled clinical trials so far published, all six, including more than 3400 patients, demonstrate decreased survival of between 1 and 10% in irradiated patients when compared with those treated by mastectomy alone."[84]

Yet, by 1980, a national survey of radiologists showed that

50% of them still radiated women following surgery for breast cancer.[85]

Either the radiologists were incompetent and not reading the medical literature, or they simply preferred to make the money, no matter that tests showed they were killing their patients.

Daniel Greenberg's "A Critical Look At Cancer Coverage" from the January-February 1975 *Columbia Journalism Review* contained the angry conclusion of one scientist regarding the radiology facts-of-life:

> "Look, when you've got 10,000 radiologists and millions of dollars worth of equipment, you give radiology treatments, even if study after study shows that a lot of it does more harm than good. What else are they going to do? They're doing what they've been trained to do."[86]

Royal Rife had determined in the 1930s that X-ray, radium and other radiation treatments produced extremely harmful effects which made the cancer of his patients more difficult to treat. Kiichiro Hasumi came to the same conclusion in the 1940s.

The destroyed tissue in the radiated area became a gathering place for the cancer virus to feast!

Rife was also able to determine the presence of cancer in 90% of his cases through a simple blood test. And he often could outline the tumor area through other methods, still ignored by the medical establishment more than 50 years later.

Studies by Irwin J. Bross, Ph.D. in the 1970s indicated that X-rays were linked to leukemia. As a result, NCI refused to renew his grant. Bross declared the cancellation was due to:

> "medical politics . . . self-interest groups protecting themselves."[87]

Bross, Director of Bio-Statistics at Roswell Park Memorial Institute for Cancer Research, accused the entire profession of radiologists from the mid-1940s to the mid-1970s (the post war generation) of committing a crime against the American people. That crime continued throughout the 1980s. It is likely to go on well into the 1990s. Bross:

> "For 30 years, radiologists in this country have been engaged in massive malpractice."[43]

A Public Broadcasting System documentary in the early 1980s, titled *The Cancer War,* included an interview with John Gofman, Ph.D., M.D., co-discoverer of 4 isotopes and 4 nuclear processes. He stated:

"My estimate is that about 94,000 cancer fatalities for the future are being induced with each year of medical diagnostic X-rays" (in the United States alone).[88]

Gofman co-authored with Egan O'Connor one of the classic studies of X-rays. Published in 1985, *X-rays: Health Effects of Common Exams* includes the following:

"Ionizing radiation, even at extremely low dose rates, breaks human chromosomes and inflicts enduring chromosomal injuries . . . a newly born child is about 300 times more sensitive than a 55-year old to induction of cancer by radiation."[89]

A 1988 book by Inlander, Levin and Weiner, utilized Gofman's and O'Connor's statistics to warn that a five-year old child was five times more susceptible to an X-ray induced cancer than a 35 year old adult while 10-year olds "may be at the greatest risk of all."[90]

Unborn fetuses apparently are in a special category. In the mid-1950s, Dr. Alice Stewart of Oxford University contacted the mothers of 1,694 children who had died of leukemia (cancer of the blood). She discovered a direct correlation between the number of times the pregnant mother had received an X-ray and the unborn child's risk of developing leukemia.

That was not surprising although the scientific facts were original. What was shocking was something else Dr. Stewart discovered. As described by Joel Griffiths and Richard Ballantine in *Silent Slaughter:*

"Stewart also found that pelvic X-rays given years *before* the mother became pregnant could predispose her child to get cancer."[91]

This caused a furor among physicians and radiologists. They bitterly dismissed the evidence for the next ten years. Then, in 1966, the National Cancer Institute published a study involving *19 million people*. It confirmed Stewart's earlier study—"X-rays given during pregnancy increase the cancer mortality in children," explained Griffiths and Ballantine. The NCI study also confirmed that pelvic X-rays given to mothers *years before* they became pregnant dramatically increased the chance of their children getting cancer!

In 1970, Dr. Alice Stewart published her second study. It included all children in Britain who died of cancer between 1943 and 1965. Griffiths and Ballantine:

> "According to Stewart's figures, the dose of a few hundred millirods from a single X-ray picture produced a 20 percent increase in cancer risk."[91]

One of the world's leading experts on low-level radiation is Dr. Ernest Sternglass, Ph.D., Professor Emeritus, Radiation Physics, University of Pittsburgh School of Medicine. He argues that low-level radiation from nuclear power plants and Chernobyl-type accidents *over a period of time* are deadlier than X-rays. Citing scientific discoveries by Dr. Segi at Tohoku University in Japan and others, Sternglass concluded that radiation pollution in the environment threatened our very existence. "If the immune system suddenly fails," he warned, "people develop cancers in terrible numbers."[92]

So how could any responsible physician or hospital center, given the abundant knowledge available on radiation, recommend radiation as a *treatment* for cancer? Memorial Sloan-Kettering Cancer Center in New York spent $4.5 million on new radiation equipment in 1980, long after the critical studies of the 1970s were completed. Memorial Sloan-Kettering *emphasized* radiation for the *majority* of its cancer patients throughout the 1980s. Why?

The answer is simple. Dr. Samuel Hellman, a radiation advocate, was in charge of their cancer treatment program. With NCI's former director, Dr. Vincent DeVita, Jr. scheduled to replace Dr. Hellman at Memorial Sloan-Kettering, it was likely that cancer treatment would shift from an emphasis on radiation to an emphasis on chemotherapy.

Dr. Hellman was scheduled to become Director of the University of Chicago Medical School. The citizens and political leaders of Illinois might be wise to seek some "objective" records regarding the survival of cancer patients at New York's Memorial Sloan-Kettering during Dr. Hellman's reign.

It might be educational to evaluate in a public forum the treatment given under Hellman's direction during his years in power. Cross-examination by experts opposed to radiation might be a valuable experience for both the good doctor Hellman and the citizens of Illinois.

According to the *New York Times,* 70% of the cancer patients treated at Memorial Sloan-Kettering in 1978-79 were given radiation treatment!

Even the "safe" levels of radiation are suspect. A cell line isolated in 1957 and named T-1 was the basis for numerous experimental research projects involving radiation doses. Only in 1980 was it discovered that T-1 had been contaminated by a particularly virulent cancer cell line known as HeLa which in laboratory experiments had been exposed to radiation, possibly producing substantial immunity to radiation. Michael Gold's 1981 book *A Conspiracy of Cells* warned:

> "Much of what was known about the harm inflicted on human cells by radiation and much of what influenced safety standards and guidelines to radiation exposure, was apparently based on experiments with T-1."[93]

Ben Fitzgerald's 1953 Senate report also included the intriguing fact that earlier studies at Memorial Sloan-Kettering had determined radiation was deadly. Somehow, despite the conclusive findings in the late 1940s and early 1950s, the radiation advocates had got their way. Fitzgerald declared:

> "There is a report from another source in which Dr. Feinblatt, for 6 years pathologist of the Memorial (Sloan-Kettering) Hospital, New York, reported that the Memorial Hospital had originally given X-ray and radium treatment before and after radical operations for breast malignancy. These patients did not long survive, so X-ray and radium were given after surgery only. These patients lived a brief time only, and after omitting all radiation, patients lived the longest of all. . ."[2]

In 1978, the Office of Technology Assessment, an arm of the United States Congress, stated that only 10% to 20% of all medical procedures had been shown to be efficacious in controlled trials. Radiation, used on millions of people, appears to fall into that category, and despite scientific evidence revealing its dangers, the army of radiologists ensures that the practice will continue—as long as uninformed patients exist and political officials fail to protect the innocent against the organized unions of physicians and radiologists.

The fact that Memorial Sloan-Kettering ignored studies which proved radiation's danger should not be surprising. Memorial Sloan-Kettering Cancer Center has a long history of burying studies and punishing researchers whose conclusions contradict the financial interests of the institution or the powerful officials at the top, many of whom have direct links to the ACS and NCI.

Item: In November 1962, Dr. John J. Harris, one of the senior scientists at MSK, was fired for co-authoring an article with the aforementioned Dr. Lawrence Burton.[48, 59]

Item: In the middle 1970s, biochemist Kanematsu Sugiura conducted tests on laetrile which produced positive results. So did scientists Dr. Lloyd Schoen and Dr. Elizabeth Smockett. Yet Sloan-Kettering officials told the press that laetrile was worthless. The true test results emerged only after dissident staff members leaked the results.[43]

Item: In 1975, MSK examined the delicate political issue of pleomorphic bacteria as a cause of cancer. This was what Glover and Deaken, Rife, Crofton and others such as Canada's Gruner had proved in the 1920s and 1930s. It had been further verified as a cause of cancer by Dr. Livingston-Wheeler, Alexander-Jackson, Seibert, Diller and still others in the 1950s and 1960s. Finally, MSK studied the issue in 1975. The results confirmed the earlier investigators. MSK dismissed its own project which obtained the results it was supposedly seeking! The excuse given was that the positive results must have resulted from outside contamination![25]

Eustace Mullins is an ardent foe of what he calls the Medical Monopoly and its international banking masters. He considers it a death threat to the American nation's freedom and democratic institutions, and identifies Memorial Sloan-Kettering as the linchpin of the New York-based cancer conspiracy. Mullins writes:

94

"The Temple of the modern method of cancer treatment in the United States is the Memorial Sloan-Kettering Cancer Institute in New York. Its high priests are the surgeons and researchers at this center. . . .

"The governing board of Memorial Sloan-Kettering Cancer Institute, called the Board of Managers, reads like a financial statement of the various Rockefeller holdings. . . .

"The Memorial Sloan-Kettering Cancer Center continues to be the most 'fashionable' charity among the New York socialites. . . .

"This institution receives $70 million a year from various tax exempt foundations . . . which means the American taxpayer is subsidizing all of this research. One hundred and thirty fulltime scientists are doing research at the Center, all 345 physicians at the Center are also heavily involved in research. And what are the results of all this activity? A continued reliance on the now antiquated 'cut, slash and burn' techniques. . . .

"While wedded to the ritual observation of these expensive, painful and futile procedures, the 'Scientists' at Sloan-Kettering maintain a resolute phalanx of opinion denouncing various wholistic procedures. . . ."[83]

Memorial Sloan-Kettering Cancer Center's budget now exceeds $335 million per year. In 1987, *each* patient *averaged* more than 6 X-Ray examinations and 4 radiation treatments.

The largest manufacturer of chemotherapy drugs is Bristol-Myers, controlling more than 50% of the U.S. market. The Chairman of the Board of Bristol-Myers is Richard Gelb. He is Vice-Chairman of the Board of Memorial Sloan-Kettering Cancer Center, an obvious and especially unethical conflict-of-interest. The other Vice-Chairman at Memorial Sloan-Kettering Cancer Center is James D. Robinson III, Chairman of the Board of American Express. He is also a Director of Bristol-Myers. And Gelb is a Director of the New York Times, perhaps insuring that the nation's most powerful newspaper will not expose the cancer industry's "dirty laundry" to its ruling class readers. A New York Times front page series on the cancer conspiracy could signal the beginning of the end and alert the power people in Washington, D.C. If only the New York Times had the courage and the patriotism.

Ralph Moss, the former assistant director of public affairs

at Memorial Sloan-Kettering Cancer Center explicitly described the cancer center/drug company "connection" in his 1989 book *The Cancer Industry:*

> "In the 1980s Memorial Sloan-Kettering Cancer Center . . . developed particularly close links with the drug industry . . . the payment for these services is usually made by arranging to split the royalties on any patents that are developed . . .
>
> "Memorial Sloan-Kettering was the prototype for all the comprehensive cancer centers. Its enormous influence and prestige serves as an amplification mechanism for this group, spreading their decisions, ripplelike, to cancer centers around the world . . .
>
> "In effect, the Memorial Sloan-Kettering Cancer Center board is a very exclusive club, which meets regularly to discuss and take actions that have repercussions for the majority of Americans. Meeting in private, keeping a low profile, they are accountable to no one but themselves for the policy decisions they make."

Dr. Robert C. Atkins, one of the most outspoken advocates of alternative and complementary medicine, and an opponent of the kind of medicine practiced at Memorial Sloan-Kettering, contends that orthodox cancer specialists are not even conducting the tests which would prove the damage they are doing with traditional radiation and chemotherapy.

> "Incredible as it may seem, most oncologists are willing to bring the immune system from normal to near zero without drawing a single immune profile (blood test). The simple white cell and platelet counts that they order just do not give adequate information. If you have a doctor who will give radiation therapy or chemotherapy without checking your immune system, you could be in for real trouble unnecessarily."[94]

When the hard changes come, and the new medicine replaces the old, when a new generation of leaders turns a critical eye on the cancer industry, and when the leaders of the AMA, FDA, NCI and ACS are found guilty of crimes against humanity, then the key people at Memorial Sloan-Kettering Cancer Center (MSKCC) should receive the same verdict of history:

"Guilty of Crimes Against Humanity."

Chapter Eight
# AIDS and Cancer

*"Drugs, alone, adulterated, or in combinations, can cause symptoms we call AIDS. No virus necessary."*
Jon Rappoport, AIDS INC.[95]

Many of the top scientists at NCI and affiliated university research centers are the same people who were the "stars" of the war on cancer in the 1970s. Searching for a virus as the cause of cancer in the 1970s, they easily switched to AIDS when it became a hot topic. Robert Gallo of NCI and Max Essex of Harvard are two of the best known. Of course, during the 70s virus hunt, no one bothered to attempt replicating Rife's 1930s studies which certainly isolated the cancer virus. (Between 1965 and 1977, NCI spent $766 million searching for the cancer virus and couldn't find it even though Rife had done it for them in 1933! And had offered to show them how to find it in 1954. He was still available until his death in 1971 but was totally ignored by the NCI "hotshots".)

When AIDS finally gained public attention in the early 1980s, it was natural that the virus hunters would attempt to isolate an AIDS virus, and, perhaps more significant, attempt to prove AIDS was caused by a virus. If AIDS was a non-virus disease, money and prestige would go elsewhere. It is so important to realize that the virus hunters had made a career out of their technical skills and knowledge. They had failed to find the cause of and a cure for cancer. But AIDS offered them a new opportunity for recognition.

In 1982, Dr. Robert Gallo of NCI was put in charge of finding the cause of AIDS.

On February 4, 1983, the AIDS virus was photographed for the first time in Paris, France. Dr. Luc Montagnier, director of viral oncology at the Pasteur Institute, was its discoverer, not Robert Gallo. A picture of the virus and an article appeared in the prestigious U.S. journal, *Science,* on May 20, 1983.

In July and September 1983, the Pasteur Institute sent samples to Gallo's laboratory outside Washington, D.C. The Pasteur Institute also filed patents on a test to determine whether people had the virus. The British patent was filed in September 1983 and the U.S. patent in December 1983.

On April 23, 1984, Gallo announced he had discovered the AIDS virus. An article appeared in the May 4, 1984 issue of *Science.* Gallo also filed a U.S. patent on April 23, 1984. This was *one year* after the French announcement of the discovery of the AIDS virus.

The U.S. Patent Office approved Gallo's patent on May 28, 1985. It ignored the French claim, filed four months prior to Gallo's and based on the same virus! The U.S. government then began receiving royalties on the Gallo AIDS test.

Meanwhile, scientists began complaining that the French virus and Gallo's virus were virtually identical. Gallo began making excuses that errors had occurred in his labs, but the scientific community began questioning Gallo's scientific integrity.

As the British journal, *New Scientist,* reported in February 1987:

> "The chances of collecting two almost identical samples of the AIDS virus are very slender, especially if they were collected several years apart. But this is just what Gallo claims."[96]

The French soon filed a legal protest. Eventually the U.S. and French governments came to a political agreement in which Gallo and Montagnier were deemed "co-discoverers" and the royalties were assigned to an international AIDS research organization. It was the most obvious of political cover-ups.

Abraham Karpas, a virologist at the University of Cambridge in England, accused Gallo of putting personal glory ahead of people's lives. By misleading researchers into thinking the AIDS virus was linked to earlier viruses that Gallo had discovered, instead of recognizing Montagnier's achievement,

Gallo had sacrificed innocent people. Karpas told the British journal, *New Scientist:*

> "A full year was wasted. In that time many lives could have been saved, many infections could have been prevented. Gallo's preoccupation . . . led many people in the wrong direction at a critical stage in AIDS research."[96]

By 1988, Gallo was still putting forth the preposterous propaganda that his emphasis in 1983 on the wrong virus (HTLV-1) contributed to the discovery of the AIDS virus (HIV). This is blatant nonsense, as many scientists recognize. Gallo's lofty position at NCI enabled him to push scientific attention in a direction which, if correct, would have brought him personal glory. But five years after being proved wrong, he still didn't have the moral courage to admit it. Gallo wrote in the October 1988 *Scientific American:*

> "That hypothesis, as it turned out, was wrong. Nevertheless, it was fruitful, because it stimulated the search that led to the correct solution."[97]

It didn't stimulate any search in the right direction. The AIDS virus had been identified by the French earlier in the year, been published in a leading American scientific journal, been presented at an important scientific convention . . . and been thoroughly ignored because American scientists were following Gallo's lead.

In November 1989, journalist John Crewdson of the Chicago Tribune finally broke the American media blackout concerning Gallo's questionable discovery of HIV, the so-called AIDS virus. Then in March 1990, Crewdson and the Chicago Tribune uncovered and published the revelation that a secret government study four years earlier in late 1985 indicated Gallo "was not the discoverer of the AIDS virus."

High officials at NCI had known all along but they covered it up!

The real, deeper, political issue is not Gallo's questionable acts regarding the discovery of the AIDS virus, but his domination of the public forum. If the HIV virus is NOT the cause of what is called AIDS, then Gallo's silencing of opponents, control of research money, and insistence that he is right (and his critics wrong) amounts to a monumental example of scientific tyranny and death for millions worldwide.

Essentially there are two views. The official or orthodox view is that AIDS is caused by the HIV virus discovered by Montagnier and Gallo. The HIV virus infects the macrophages which produce more virus. The virus then destroys the T cells. As the immune system breaks down, opportunistic infection such as pneumocystis carinii pneumonia (called simply pneumocystis or PCP) and Kaposi's sarcoma (KS) lead to inevitable death. The AIDS virus doesn't cause death in most cases. It weakens or destroys the immune system, whereupon other infections, primarily PCP or KS, cause death. Montagnier stated in the December 1988 *OMNI* that because they can handle the opportunistic infections better now than at the outset of AIDS, they observe "more people dying of the AIDS virus itself."[98]

The second view is the "underground" view—not reported to any degree in the press, not discussed in scientific journals, not funded for research, whispered among eminent researchers but rarely with any public use of their names. This view is that there is no proof that the HIV virus causes AIDS. It may simply be a minor virus which the body can handle. This might mean that if a person is tested "positive" for HIV antibodies, it means little and certainly not death. It might simply mean that your immune system's antibodies are handling the virus rather well just as they handle many others. (This is the principle of vaccines.)

The underground view, if true, points of course to a monstrous scandal. If those officially in charge of the AIDS war are wrong, have taken all that money for research, and have taken the country and indeed the world down a deadend path, while denying the money to various orthodox and alternative treatments which could have saved millions of lives, then these American medical experts—Gallo, Essex, Hazeltine, Broder, Fauci, etc.—are guilty not only of a monumental error but of a monumental crime. If, to enhance their reputations or fortunes, they deliberately ignored possibilities other than the one involving their specialty, they have not only failed in their public responsibility, they have committed manslaughter on a massive scale—even if it was not consciously done.

For example, suppose that having antibodies to the HIV virus is of no real importance. This would mean that AZT (the only authorized treatment) is being given to healthy people, thus destroying their immune systems and eventually causing their deaths. If this is the case, then those responsible—again Gallo, Essex, Hazeltine, Broder and Fauci (the key five although there are many others)—have much to account for to the people who put their lives in the hands of these five men. AZT is being irresponsibly used by many doctors, as reported in the December 21, 1987 *New York Times*. AZT is *not* being given only to terminal AIDS patients but also to many who simply test positive for antibodies to the HIV virus. This is why the questions concerning the scientific policies and the censorship of alternative views go far, far beyond careerism and gaining grant money for one's own government or university empire. They go to the heart of morality. And scientific integrity.

The outstanding book in the field describing the alternative view on AIDS is *AIDS Inc.,* by Jon Rappoport. It is available for $13.95 plus $2.00 postage (total $15.95) from: Human Energy Press, Suite D, 370 West San Bruno Avenue, San Bruno, CA 94066. If you, the reader, read but one book on AIDS in your lifetime, make it this one. It may save your life.

Rappoport interviewed many, many scientists while researching his book. He read many, many scientific journals. And he asked the questions which the scientists and doctors in charge of the AIDS war should have asked but did not.

His definition of AIDS is simple and worth remembering:

"What is AIDS. . . . It is any form of severe immunosuppression, from any source, which then gives rise to opportunistic infections. . . .

"AIDS is merely immune-collapse followed by opportunistic infection."[95]

Simple. But then Rappoport goes on to show that drugs can cause immunosuppression. So can chemicals in our food. So can medical drugs. So can malnutrition. Read the book. PCP is caused by a protozoa. 70-80% of healthy people carry it. Drug-taking, immune-suppressing chemotherapy for cancer, a promiscuous life style—*all* of these could activate PCP, not only the vaunted HIV virus which the U.S. government has already spent hundreds of millions in defending and researching, with billions more likely to be wasted.

Kaposi's sarcoma (KS), according to Rappoport, appears to be connected to the "use of poppers in the U.S." In other words, AIDS may not be a gay disease at all, but rather a disease closely linked to drugs—medical drugs, recreational drugs and other immune-suppressing activities such as promiscuity.

In fact Rappoport and Montagnier appear to agree that AIDS is a disease of modern civilization.

From Montagnier's December 1988 *OMNI* interview:

> "The conditions of civilization have caused the epidemic. . . . We're a civilization of blood, of blood transfusions. The practice has existed for only a little over half a century and then came the so-called sexual revolution. We've created a one world environment for our germs."[98]

It is important to emphasize that Montagnier believes that the HIV virus *is* the cause of AIDS and is in fact the most sinister virus ever discovered. If he is correct, then the determined efforts by him and his American peers should be honored. But if they are wrong and simpler explanations exist, then a gigantic and tragic scam has been perpetrated. Science is supposed to be objective. It functions only if there is honest, open dialogue. This is *not* happening in the current medi-political environment. The scientists are fearful and silent.

Rappoport says simply:

> "AIDS is a drug-related phenomenon, almost across the board. Throw out the risk-groups and just look into the backgrounds of those diagnosed with AIDS and you will, in the overwhelming majority of cases, find drug abuse."[95]

In other words, it isn't "needle-sharing" that causes AIDS. It is the damned drugs the addicts take that produce immune suppression and enable the opportunistic infections to kill. Again, Rappoport:

"People whose health is compromised, but still very reversible are not being told *how* significant these drug factors are in their lives. That is criminal."[95]

You see, if the real cause of AIDS is not perceived or, if known, is covered up, then the appropriate treatments cannot be developed. Rappoport writes:

"The cure to what is called AIDS has much to do with the proposition that immune systems can be repaired. Although, in this, medicine has little experience or skill."[95]

Which brings us back to cancer and the suppression of the alternative treatments which in fact do enable immune systems to be restored.

With the NCI people in charge of the AIDS virus hunt and the "drug question" swept under the rug, drug treatment for AIDS in the hospitals can continue. Drug companies can seek their financial bonanzas (Burroughs-Wellcome being the first to cash in with the drug AZT which suppresses the immune system). Homeopathy, acupuncture and bio-electronics, modalities which had a real chance of successfully treating AIDS, have been totally ignored.

In the summer of 1984, after only 6 weeks of trials on twenty subjects, NCI organized a national trial for the drug Suramin. This was the first national AIDS trial. None of the 20 AIDS patients under observation had shown any improvement, but NCI needed to do something because of public and political pressure. The quick OK after only 6 weeks (and no results) shows how quickly the federal agencies can act if they wish to.

Suramin was a disaster. It caused severe effects on the liver, kidneys and adrenal glands. It was not a new drug, but one with a history of being dangerous. Yet the physicians in charge of the clinical trials at the five national centers didn't even test to determine the damage Suramin was doing to the patients' adrenal glands:

"One of the drug's main side effects was a malfunctioning of the adrenal glands. And somehow those administering the drug at each of the five medical centers involved in the Suramin study failed to include a simple low cost test for adrenal damage."[99]

The trial began in March 1985, even though in January 1985 NCI had already notified the participating hospitals that significant toxicity was appearing. The trial ended abruptly in December 1985 when the awful results could no longer be ignored. It was a human sacrifice. The doctors in charge at San Francisco General were severely criticized for their behavior. Ethical violations were cited. Yet Dr. Paul Volberding, Dr. Lawrence Kaplan and Dr. Walter Way all continued in their positions. Their careers were unblemished by the tragedy which occurred under their supervision. Charles Linebarger reported:

> "Patients were given double doses of Suramin without signing new consent forms. . . . Patients with chronic hepatitis, a serious liver disease, were allowed into the study and given massive doses of Suramin; the drug is known to damage healthy livers, much less diseased ones."[99]

The death toll? Of the 23 patients in the test cite at San Francisco in 1985, 20 were dead by 1988. The way they died can be directly traced to the drug they were given:

> "Some died of liver toxicity, which caused their stomachs to blow up to the size of laundry bags. Others died of AIDS infections suddenly gone crazy. . . ."[99]

Eventually AZT came along. Like Suramin, it was an old drug taken off the shelf at NCI. It became the first drug approved for general use with AIDS patients. It was first found to inhibit the AIDS virus in the laboratory in February 1985. In March 1987, it was approved as a prescription drug following a 6-month double blind clinical trial from February 1986 to September 1986. The two-year process was considered fast. Gloated NCI scientists: "We attribute this rapid development to the careful, scientific controlled process by which the clinical trials were conducted."[100]

Since the 6-month AZT trial resulted in the patients' CD4 levels returning to their *pretreatment* levels, it is astonishing that *widespread* use of AZT was allowed. A patient's CD4 level indicates how the immune system's T cells are doing against the disease. With AZT, improvement occurred, but then reverted to a pretreatment level. There was no great rationale for getting excited about AZT, especially with its toxicity. But AZT did take the pressure off the NCI scientists and was a bonanza for Burroughs-Wellcome, the drug company that stole the rights from NCI. (NCI officials admit they made "errors" with the commercial rights. In other words, they did not protect the public interest.)

Many experts now agree that the original AZT trial which resulted in FDA approval was absolutely worthless. Celia Farber's devastating 1990 exposé in *SPIN* magazine, "Sins of Omission: The AZT Scandal," made that basic fact hard to ignore:

> "the decision to approve it was based on a single study that has long been declared invalid . . . 'There was no great difference after a while,' says Dr. (Itzhak) Brook (panel chairman who voted against approval) 'between the treated and the untreated group.'
>
> "The country has been brainwashed . . . The data has all been manipulated by people who have a lot vested in AZT.
>
> "Dr. Harvey Bialy, science editor of the journal Biotechnology . . . is horrified . . . because, he insists, the claims its widespread use are based upon are false."

Dr. Joseph Sonnabend, who spent 10 years at the British National Institute for Medical Research and who edited *AIDS Research,* a respected journal in the field, told Rappoport:

> "AZT trials. . . . That trial was so wrong, so badly done. It's terrible."[95]

The man in charge of the trial was Sam Broder of NCI. Sam Broder is the new Director of the NCI and its $1.5 billion annual budget. The questions which ought to be asked about this man's performance regarding AZT and his qualifications to lead the entire national cancer program are obvious. Someday, in one form or another, they will be asked.

The history of AZT and the suppression of potentially better drugs has been courageously exposed by Bruce Nussbaum in his 1990 book, *Good Intentions: How Big Business and the*

*Medical Establishment Are Corrupting the Fight Against AIDS*.[101]

In October 1984, Sam Broder of NCI went to the drug company Burroughs Wellcome of Raleigh, North Carolina and offered to cooperate on AIDS drugs. (Broder was responsible for the Suramin fiasco.) Burroughs Wellcome took Broder to the cleaners. They took AZT, a second-rate, toxic cancer drug and sent it to Broder who got excited in February 1985 when it showed activity against the (so-called) AIDS virus in laboratory cell cultures.

Then Dr. David Barry of Burroughs-Wellcome, a former deputy director of the Division of Virology at FDA, contacted his old institution. In April 1985, he cut a special deal with Dr. Ellen Cooper who was the key administrator in approving antiviral drugs. In 3 months, all the preliminary dog, rat and other experiments were completed. In June 1985, after only *5 days* of data analysis (instead of the usual several months), Cooper permitted Broder at NCI to inject the first patient with AZT. Soon full scale trials were underway in North Carolina and at NCI.

Meanwhile, Congress had begun to pour money into AIDS research. Dr. Anthony Fauci of the National Institute of Allergy and Infectious Diseases managed to grab most of the newly allocated AIDS money for his institution. He became America's "AIDS Czar." Trouble was neither he nor anyone at his institute had any experience in managing large trials. So *hundreds of millions of dollars* went nowhere during the next three years and the entire AIDS program got clogged with AZT.

In January 1987, the critical committee decision at FDA took place which would decide whether to approve AZT for marketing. But the independent investigators on the committee were shocked to discover that the Burroughs Wellcome and Broder/NCI trials were a disgrace. They were about to *disapprove* AZT when Dr. David Barry's old boss at FDA entered the room. Subtle political pressure changed the committee's decision.

Millions of sick, desperate, dying patients were about to get AZT, a second-rate, highly toxic, essentially ineffective drug because of the old-boy network and one drug company's clever politics.

Soon Burroughs Wellcome had loaded up Anthony Fauci's AIDS drug approval committee with its own, paid, "outside" investigators. Drugs which competed with AZT were not funded or tested.

In August 1989, the committee announced the trial results for AZT used on people who were HIV positive but had no symptoms associated with AIDS. Two years of study involving thousands of people showed AZT helped stop the progression of AIDS, Fauci claimed. It was a lie. European scientists examined the same data and concluded that Anthony Fauci's "experts" were all wet! By then, a significant number of this critical AIDS committee were financially linked to Burroughs Wellcome, with at least two of the key people making video advertisements for AZT and Burroughs Wellcome—Dr. Margaret Fischl of the University of Miami and Dr. Paul Volberding of San Francisco General Hospital (of Suramin fame); Broder also appeared on video for Burroughs Wellcome, an incredible conflict-of-interest for a government public health official.

By March 1990, even the AMA Journal was questioning the use of AZT for people who showed no symptoms associated with AIDS. A separate Veterans Administration trial had proved the opposite of what the Burroughs Wellcome gang inside Fauci's government agency had sold to the public.

"the supposedly unbiased researchers who even did a Burroughs Wellcome video extolling the virtues of AZT . . . took control of the government's entire anti-AIDS effort . . . they ran all the major committees . . . which voted on every single potential anti-AIDS drug. In effect, scientists who had bet their professional careers on one drug, AZT, were put in positions to vote on other drugs that might compete with AZT . . . It was a clear institutional conflict of interest and not a single voice was raised inside the world of research, inside the National Institutes of Health or the FDA, against it.

"They were accountable to no one but themselves. They were invisible to the public eye.

"No one . . . had ever taken a serious critical look inside

the clinical trials network system. For over forty years . . . no questions were asked by any public or private body about how the Principal Investigators (PIs) went about testing new drugs on humans."[101]

The issue is a fundamental one. Will there be a democratic element in scientific and health matters, or will so-called experts impose their views? Jad Adams phrased the issue as follows in the fall of 1990 issue of *Policy Review:*

"Ultimately expert advice must be evaluated by the people who are not experts—politicians, journalists and the public. This is part of democratic life and a scientist has no more right to exclusion from public scrutiny than a treasury official.

"All expert advice affecting our lives must be subjected to abrasive doubt. In the field of the HIV theory this doubt has had a struggle to thrive in the scientific community. It needs an infusion of energy from outsiders whose only interest is to ensure that hard questions are asked and the AIDS establishment is pinned down to answer them."

Of course such a public involvement would lead necessarily to the billion dollar question: does HIV cause AIDS or, as is now being whispered in scientific back-rooms, has there been a monumental screw-up followed by a political cover-up with monstrous consequences?

In March 1987, *Cancer Research,* a prestigious journal, published an article by Dr. Peter Duesberg in which he questioned the AIDS virus theory. Duesberg, a molecular biologist at the University of California Berkeley and the co-discoverer of the first cancer gene, virtually confronted the entire AIDS establishment. He was met by silence.

Duesberg's original article was followed by subsequent pieces or interviews in *Biotechnology,* November 1987, *New Scientist,* April 28, 1988, the *Wall Street Journal* and other newspapers. Duesberg was saying "something else"—other than the virus—caused AIDS. Gallo and his supporters vehemently disagreed—for a while. Then Gallo began making strange noises, shifting, shifting, shifting. He continued to denounce and dismiss Duesberg, but then suddenly announced that he had just discovered what might be a "cofactor" in

AIDS. This is what Duesberg had been saying! A cofactor might explain why all the T4 cells are virtually destroyed in AIDS patients when laboratory tests show that the AIDS virus kills only a few T4 cells at a time.

The body's T4 cell replacements outnumber (easily) what is being destroyed in the laboratory by the AIDS virus. But a cofactor might explain the slaughter of the T4 cells and the rapid collapse of AIDS patients. Gallo wouldn't give Duesberg credit but more objective scientists were willing to recognize the validity of Duesberg's position.

Walter Gilbert, a Nobel Prize winner and Harvard professor, supported Duesberg's primary criticism:

> "He is absolutely correct in saying that no one has proven that AIDS is caused by the AIDS virus. And he is absolutely correct that the virus cultured in the laboratory may not be the cause of AIDS. There is no animal model for AIDS, and where there is no animal model, you cannot establish Koch's postulates. Peter exaggerates some of the numbers, but the basic argument is perfectly true."[103]

What all this reveals is a familiar story. The same kind of experts who have been in charge of the cancer war are dominating the AIDS war. Dr. Joseph Sonnabend told Rappoport:

> "There really is now such a thing as the AIDS establishment. It is a group which receives virtually all the grant money, it sits on important boards (such as the fund raising organization, Americans for AIDS Research). There is definitely a group, and sadly, it's not the best talent."

Sonnabend added:

> "The ones who agree HIV causes AIDS get their articles printed."[95]

Duesberg, the voice in the wilderness, was ignored or dismissed by the establishment. So Rappoport asked Duesberg what he would do if he were in charge of the national AIDS program. Duesberg's answer evoked what many, many critics of the 50-year national cancer program have determined to be the primary misstep in cancer policy: too many dollars wasted on lab research controlled by a small group of insiders, and not enough spent at the patient level. Duesberg:

"I would take AIDS research from the lab much more into the clinical situation. See what patients are showing. What are their signs. I would look at patients much more. Our instrumentation these days is so sensitive. So we have a tendency to remove ourselves from real life."

And AZT? Duesberg:

"I think AZT is the most sinister aspect of this whole business. They're killing growing (normal) cells. That's what they're doing. That's very serious business."[95]

For Montagnier, the HIV virus was sinister. For Duesberg, using AZT when the HIV virus was not known to be the cause of AIDS was sinister. One of these two eminent scientists is wrong. Many lives are on the line.

In the meantime, scientific discoveries concerning AIDS and the HIV virus continue to be announced. But no effective treatment ever results. Anything original offered from the lowly front lines is ignored and any criticism of the experts, even from one of their own, results in furious denouncements or silence.

Even more disturbing is the possibility that Gallo and the medical elite's virus hunt has misled the entire American nation and the world as to the real threat—that pesticides and prescription drugs are the real cause of AIDS. Rappoport presented the following, frightening scenario during a television interview:

"Pesticides and pharmaceuticals are quite dangerous. . . . You are opening the door to a large amount of immune suppression plus opportunistic infections among people. . . . You can bring about the same identical pattern of AIDS by the use of chemicals. . . . AIDS is going to become a smokescreen for whatever is happening in the Third World. . . . Huge use of pesticides. . . . Dumping of drugs that are too dangerous to use in this country. . . . We are presenting a definition of AIDS in the Third World as being identical to starvation and malnutrition. Politically this opens the door to . . . a form of political repression that needs no ideology. . . . Declare Medical States of Emergency. Armaments of the modern priest-

110

hood which is 'White Coats and Science'. . . . You might be surprised to see how fast it could spread."[104]

One of the main issues presented by Rappoport and the scientists he has interviewed is that science in the AIDS war has been sacrificed for medical politics to a degree that is unprecedented. Rappoport discusses how drugs were *not* examined as the cause of AIDS, how the records of the AZT trials were altered later, and how views critical of the "official" HIV policy were censored.

An interesting little book which presents a similar picture of political shenanigans driving medical policies, this time not at NCI but the Centers for Disease Control, appeared in October 1988. Its author, Gus G. Sermos, worked as a Public Health Advisor and AIDS Researcher at the Centers for Disease Control (CDC) for a number of years. He described in his book how CDC officials did not want to investigate certain aspects of the AIDS epidemic. Public health appeared not to be their primary concern. Rather, being politically correct seemed more important. Sermos declares that many lives and much money have been wasted:

> "What happens if the people you trust and count on to study the spread of diseases and epidemics lie to you? What happens when public health officials decide they do not want to find out all they can about the agent, host, and environmental factors? . . . Bodies and money are what happen. More people become infected; more people die; and the costs of the AIDS epidemic continue to accelerate."[105]

In April 1990 an interview of Peter Duesberg by journalist Russell Schoch appeared in the magazine *California Monthly*. Schoch opened by summarizing some of the most disturbing "problems" with the orthodox view that AIDS was a new disease spread by a new virus. Among the items was the one the NCI people and the mainstream media kept ignoring:

> "If HIV acted like a conventional virus, it would by now have spread far beyond its original points of attack. The virus would be random in the population, as was predicted in 1983 when it was discovered; this, however, has not come to pass."

Duesberg had not wavered in the three years since he had gone public against the conventional wisdom. If anything his

111

position had strengthened since reports had appeared which showed some patients with Kaposi's Sarcoma (KS) were free of the HIV virus. How could patients with one of the two primary AIDS diseases not have any sign of the accepted *cause* of AIDS? Duesberg's answer: "That's usually the kiss of death in an etiology study: if you can get the same disease without the agent, the agent can't be the cause."

Duesberg, like others, was more and more horrified by the growing, indiscriminant use of AZT when there was no solid proof that HIV caused AIDS or that AZT stopped HIV. To Duesberg, AIDS was a "drug epidemic associated with malnutrition." And AZT was "essentially chemotherapy . . . it kills cells . . . I think there is no rational basis for treating any AIDS patient with AZT . . . we are about to kill off, intoxicate, 50,000 people with AZT. That's the number now taking AZT. And that's the same number of people we lost in Vietnam."

Celia Farber's 1990 *SPIN* article included the little reported fact that a major independent study in France of AZT (on more patients than the original FDA study) determined that "after a few months . . . AZT was completely ineffective."

Dr. Sonnabend complained to Farber: "We're being held hostage by second-rate scientists . . . This is such shoddy science it's hard to believe nobody is protesting. Damned cowards. The name of the game is protect your grant, don't open your mouth. It's all about money."

Meanwhile, alternative treatments in America already are being combated with legal harassment. In the name of protecting the patients, and scientific procedures, the dying are denied the right to choose for themselves therapies which, while "unproven," might open the way to breakthroughs. Since these alternative therapies will never be tested anyway because the boss scientists aren't interested (and if they did work they would likely be suppressed), the utter cruelty, injustice and criminality of the system are apparent.

The FDA, according to Commissioner Frank Young, defines "quackery, or health fraud, as the promotion of a false or unproven product or therapy for profit."

The word "unproven" is the key. Any "unproven" therapy

is subject to criminal prosecution. Whatever the authorities ignore, despite overwhelming evidence, is "unproven." Alice-in-Wonderland rules, standards and laws operate here—in direct contradiction to the body of criminal law in the United States.

On May 21, 1987, the Attorney General of California began investigating AIDS consumer fraud and quackery. It was the first state action to punish those offering any unconventional, non-FDA approved treatment. It was not surprising that such an action was initiated in California. After the drug company-sponsored "Coordinating Conference on Health Information" assumed a lower profile following numerous protests against the government agencies involved in unconstitutional harass-ment and crackdowns on those threatening the drug monopoly (1964-1974), many officials of the CCHI quietly moved into key positions in the California State Board of Health. Califor-nia being a hot bed of new ideas and alternative health, it was the logical place for the suppressors to conduct low-publicity actions against innovations dangerous to the medical pow-ers.[83]

Senator Quentin L. Copp, San Francisco, appears to be the leading legislator in the California Senate who serves the interests of the drug/AMA syndicate.

Still, AIDS patients kept dying. No treatments sanctioned by the medical hierarchy worked. And more and more protest was building, with Congress and FDA getting the heat. Some nifty excuse-making and compromises were needed. On July 14, 1988, the *Los Angeles Times* reported that FDA Commis-sioner Frank Young had testified before Congress, arguing that only one or two of 320 compounds now being tested against AIDS would be "successful therapies" by 1991. He insisted on FDA's slow procedures being maintained.

Within weeks, Commissioner Young had reversed his pos-ition and announced that AIDS patients could import foreign drugs which hadn't been approved by FDA. However, Amer-ican firms would have to play by the old rules. *The Wall Street Journal* of July 26, 1988 ridiculed such a double standard. Safety, effectiveness and quality control were removed for "patients bootlegging drugs into the U.S." Those unfortunate enough to have no access to foreign drugs would have safety, effectiveness and quality control, but no alternatives.

Then, in another shift on August 1, 1988, FDA began blocking a foreign AIDS drug from Canada. Why? The company making the drug had *promoted* it. That was prohibited. If someone suffering from AIDS found out about a foreign drug, then they could legally import it. But if the foreign company *promoted* the drug, it would be banned. The FDA seemed to be demonstrating a new form of institutional schizophrenia. Previously, the pressure came from the higher-ups and FDA willingly obliged. Now pressure was coming from below via the patients and from above via the drug companies who didn't like the special rules for the foreign competitors. So FDA thrust first in one direction, then another. It would have been hilarious if the human suffering weren't so evident.

On August 15, 1988, FDA relaxed its rules on effectiveness for one domestic drug company. It allowed a drug, trimetrexate, which showed no indication of being effective, to be used by some AIDS patients. The drug was made by Warner-Lambert of New Jersey, whose former president, Elmer Bobst, had helped reorganize the American Cancer Society. But the FDA's latest shift raised an obvious question. If such a change could be permitted for AIDS patients, why not for cancer patients? The *total* number of deaths from AIDS by May 1988 was 34,526. That many people died from cancer *every month*.

On December 22, 1987, Dr. Anthony Fauci, director of the national AIDS program, made the cancer-AIDS merger official:

> "The model for our work is cancer treatment, where we attempt to assemble a potent mixture of drugs."

Dr. John Cairns' assessment of chemotherapy's 2% to 3% effectiveness in the cancer war, so carefully presented in the November 1985 *Scientific American,* was now conveniently ignored by the press, the NCI officials and the political representatives elected by the people to guard their interest.

So AIDS treatment and a hope for a cure appeared to be caught in the same vise as cancer treatment and the long-promised cure—FDA barriers to anything innovative, loopholes for the big drug companies (Warner-Lambert had a net income for the first nine months of 1988 of $262 million while Merck had $900 million), NCI dominated "research" . . . and all the other indications of a medical monopoly killing people. All of it was legal. All of it was sanctioned. And most of it was never mentioned by the press.

The game had become so blatant a racket that the leading non-profit, fund-raising AIDS organization, the American Foundation for AIDS Research (AMFAR), was headed by Mathilde Krim. Remember Mathilde Krim?

Krim was Mary Lasker's buddy who helped start the "war on cancer" in 1970-71 and whose enthusiasm for interferon in 1979 led to the third major American Cancer Society raid on the U.S. Treasury in the 70s decade. By 1985, Krim had decided to surrender her position as head of the Interferon Lab at Memorial Sloan-Kettering in order to initiate the "war on AIDS." The new AIDS foundation (AMFAR) headquarters was just down the street from the American Cancer Society headquarters.

And in November 1988, the FDA approved the use of interferon for AIDS patients with Kaposi's sarcoma. One had to wonder whether all the millions of dollars of warehoused interferon from the 1979-1981 period was still available. Dr. William Hazeltine, one of the AIDS top five, had suggested that babies who tested as HIV positive be given a week of AZT, then a week of interferon. The FDA decision merely made such a practice legitimate. The Mathilde Krim-interfe-ron-AIDS link was, of course, just a coincidence.

Even worse, Dr. Ellen Cooper of FDA had insisted that drug trials with babies required a placebo control . . . which meant *half the babies had to die* to satisfy Cooper's distorted, immoral and fundamentally *disturbed* view of science. "These experiments always required that . . . the proof be death . . . dead babies."[101]

Rappaport asked Dr. Joseph Sonnabend about the use of interferon for AIDS patients. Sonnabend had done early research on interferon and AIDS. He replied:

"No good is coming of it. I asked an interferon researcher how they could continue to give AIDS patients this when it

115

had such clear immunosuppressive properties. He said, well, the drug companies had such huge unsold stocks of recombinant interferon."[95]

So the curse of Mary Lasker and Mathilde Krim continued.

Hold onto your wallets, America. All that money being authorized by Congress and being petitioned from the public by Krim's AMFAR for "AIDS research, information and treatment" is going to the same kind of people who ran the "war on cancer" and grew rich at the American Cancer Society.

> "Those who eat their fill speak to the hungry
> Of wonderful times to come."
>
> Brecht

Bruce Nussbaum's brilliant book *Good Intentions* describes the real scandal-horror-killing machine which must be dismantled and replaced, not only in dealing with AIDS but also with cancer.

> "It is a polite fiction that the NIH (National Institutes of Health) does public health. It will receive about $9 billion from Congress in 1990 to do medical research that is supposed to benefit the public. Three-quarters of it will be sent to principal investigators (PIs) in their elite academic institutions around the country . . . their experiments have little to do with either health or the public. They test drugs by private pharmaceutical companies for personal gain, for money that goes to their universities, and for power.
>
> "The . . . AIDS Program . . . billions of taxpayer dollars have disappeared into the private projects of a handful of scientists who insist they know what is best for the health of the country. It is simply not true; they don't."[101]

In June 1990, Luc Montagnier announced that HIV was a benign virus and did not cause AIDS by itself. The American media totally ignored the bombshell. People continued to get AZT for a virus that may do them no harm. On December 23, 1990, journalist Elinor Burkett finally described the cover-up in the Miami Herald. The rest of the American media continued its blackout of the truth about AIDS.

Chapter Nine
# The Cancer Microbe

*"Most microbial diseases today are caused by microbes which . . . are present all the time in the body of normal individuals . . . they become the cause of a disease when some disturbance occurs which upsets the equilibrium."*
Rene Dubos, renowned microbiologist[25]

Modern 20th century medicine has been based on a fundamental error. That error can be traced to the famous 19th century chemist Louis Pasteur (1822-1895). Simply expressed, the error is the "germ theory." According to this model, microbes (germs) enter a body and disease results. Vaccines and various chemicals are used to destroy the germ or prevent it from doing its damage. What is conveniently ignored is that Pasteur denounced his own theory on his deathbed. He stated, "Bernard is right. The microbe is nothing. The environment is all important."

Claude Bernard (1813-1878) was a French physiologist who claimed that the seeds of disease—the germs or microbes— would not grow (and cause disease) unless the "terrain" or environment in the body was conducive. This cause and effect relationship emphasized by Bernard is ignored by most modern researchers who, introducing alien elements in their laboratories (artificial terrain), fail to emphasize sufficiently the basic processes of disease in the body.

Certainly deadly germs exist or can be created which even the healthiest human cannot withstand. But these infectious microbes are not the problem for the average person. With degenerative diseases such as cancer and possibly a great deal of AIDS, Bernard's emphasis on the inner environment is most significant.

Bernard's *An Introduction to the Study of Experimental Medicine* was published by Dover Publications, New York, in 1957. Originally published in France in 1865, "it remains a classic text on physiology, and application of the scientific in medicine," according to one determined biological theorist.[106]

The chief contemporary rival of Pasteur was Antoine Bechamp (1816-1908). He is known to have provided Pasteur with ideas and techniques which Pasteur blatantly stole. Pasteur was politically powerful, his own erroneous notions commercially profitable, and his opposition to Bechamp legendary. Pasteur was able to force Bechamp's exile from scientific circles. However, Bechamp's discoveries were never entirely lost and in each succeeding generation a few dedicated researchers have carried Bechamp's work forward.

Bechamp identified tiny moving bodies which he named *microzymas* (also called microzymes). According to Bechamp, these particles were everywhere and were indestructible. They formed the living tissue of plants and animals. And they also were the seeds from which bacteria came into being and destruction of the body, through disease, occurred. When the body died, the bacteria returned to their earlier *microzyme* or *seed* form. Modern day researchers consider the microzymes as preceding DNA.

Monica Bryant summarized Bechamp's theory as follows in the March 1986 *Journal of Alternative Medicine:*

> "Bechamp believed that there were small particles, 'granulations moléculaires', which were present in all living matter and were indestructible and eternal. He named these primal units *microzymes* and they marked the transition between non-living and living matter. . . . For Bechamp disease was seen to originate from *within* the body, as opposed to Pasteur's view that all diseases were caused by bacteria which invaded the body from the outer environment and came from pre-existing bacteria . . . Bechamp's view emphasizes the fact that pathogenic microorganisms are not the *cause* of disease, but rather the *secondary manifestation* of a state of toxicity in the body."[107]

These "seeds," according to Bechamp and later researchers, thus served to maintain health and orchestrate adaptation. But they also were the means by which the body's inner "terrain" was altered into a disease state, leading to death. Some kind of cellular metabolic irritation altered the seeds or microzymes in their interaction with its terrain. The seeds take charge of the terrain, modifying it to suit a change in the seeds' purpose. As John Mattingly has written, "The microzymes had the power of breaking down the tissues and the very cells of which they once formed a part. In the process of doing so they would evolve into bacteria; but when the work of the bacteria was completed and there was nothing more on which they could live, they would revert again to microzymes."[106]

Bechamp had found microzymes alive and healthy in the remains of ancient corpses.

In its destructive phase, the seed first became a fungus. It is recognized that mycology—the study of fungi—and particularly mycosis, the diseases caused by fungi, have been largely ignored by 20th century medicine. The separation of mycology and bacteriology—or fungi and bacteria in their relation to disease—is one of the tragic developments of 20th century medicine.

Rife's cure for cancer in the 1930s was based on scientific work which proved that a particular fungus could be transformed into a cancer-causing bacterium the size of a virus. Because he could destroy the bacterium and the fungus, Rife was able to reverse the cancer process.

It is important to emphasize the *size* and *enormous number* of the microbes which come forth from the microzymes when the environment or terrain is conducive for the destructive phase to begin.

From Peter Farb's *Living Earth:*

"Even in a teaspoon of soil from the temperate regions, there may be five billion bacteria . . . a million protozoa, and 200,000 algae and fungi. These crowds of micro-organisms carry on such a fierce activity on each acre that they expend an amount of energy equal to 10,000 human beings living and working there."[108]

From *Business Week,* September 22, 1986:

"Fifteen years and $13 billion after the declared war on cancer, the prognosis is still grim. Of the nearly 1 million Americans diagnosed with cancer each year, only half will be alive in 5 years. Surgery, radiation and highly toxic drugs all tend to fail for a stunningly simple reason: a tumor the size of your thumb has 1 billion malignant cells in it. Even if a treatment gets 99.9% of them, a million remain to take root all over again."[109]

According to Roy Rife's laboratory notes in the 1930s, the cancer causing microbe was so small that if 500,000 of them were put side by side, the total size would be one inch!

Bechamp regarded his "seeds" as a necessary anatomical element which under certain "conditions of disease" evolved into disease-causing forms. As the terrain of the body was disturbed from its healthy condition, disease followed. Not because a germ invaded. But because of a shock or accident. Because of the natural aging process. Or because of the mind influencing negative body states. Or something else.

Roy Rife proved in his 1930s laboratory that by "altering the environment," he could change a harmless bacteria into a deadly one, and then reverse it again.

"We have proved that it is the chemical constituents . . . of the virus under observation which enact upon the unbalanced cell metabolism of the body to produce any disease that may occur. We have in many instances produced all the symptoms of the disease chemically without the innoculation of any virus or bacteria in the tissues of experimental animals.

"We have classified the entire category of pathogenic bacteria into 10 groups. Any organism within its group can be readily changed to any other organism within the ten groups depending upon the media with which it is fed and grown. For example, with a pure culture of baccillus coli, by altering the media as little as two parts per million by volume, we can change that micro-organism in 36 hours to a bacillus typhosis showing every known laboratory test. . . .

"Further controlled alterations of the media will end up with the virus of poliomelitis or tuberculosis or cancer as desired, and then, if you please, alter the media again and change the micro-organism back to a bacillus coli."[110]

Doctor Royal Lee of the Lee Foundation for Nutritional Research in Milwaukee, a friend and associate of Rife, summarized Rife's biological discovery as follows:

"Rife showed that there are only about ten different classes of germs, within each class conversion from one form to another is a matter of environment."

What Rife was doing in modern terms was *communicating* with microbes. By altering the environment, disease states were reversed. Modern bio-electronic instruments, using healthy homeopathic frequencies sent electronically, also can signal or induce the body back into a healthy state. A few people claim to be able to do this through conscious mental processes. In time, a large proportion of humanity may be able to do the same.

Daniel Koshland of the University of California Berkeley has demonstrated that bacteria can think. They remember and make decisions.[111]

Common to a number of researchers is the idea of non-physical informational transfers between cells. Candice Pert and Michael Ruff, well-known for their peptide studies, think of consciousness as being "located in every cell in the body."[112]

Robert O. Becker, author of *The Body Electric,* suggests that this future direction can be scientifically understood, scientifically validated, and individually learned:

"I predict that research on this system will eventually let us learn to control pain, healing, and growth with our minds alone, substantially reducing the need for physicians."[113]

Brendan O'Regan of the consciousness studying Noetic Institute noted that negative expectations can have stunning effects which potentially alter the premises of so-called double blind studies. He describes the results of one clinical trial as follows:

"There is another intriguing example from the *World Journal of Surgery,* which reported on the test of a new kind of chemotherapy in 1983. As is often the case in such tests, there was an experimental group that received the chemotherapy, and a control group that received a sugar pill or an inert substance. One of the effects of chemotherapy that we're familiar with is hair loss—so people *expect* to lose their hair when given chemotherapy. In this study 30 percent of the control group—given placebos—lost their hair. That's a very physical effect. . . . Given these physical effects of placebos, one wonders what is going on. There must be complex pathways between mind and body and indeed belief systems."[114]

To return briefly to Bechamp, it is his microzyme theory and its emphasis on the inner environment that is the basis for questioning the dominant medical model governing treatment. Throughout this century, the scientific hierarchy has ignored research which proves that bacteria can change their size and shape, becoming the size of a virus. Whether a virus is only part of a cycle involving bacteria is not the question. Bacteria the size of a virus exist, yet are ignored by the dominant school of thought. Rife's work and the work of many others suggest that Bechamp's theory deserves serious, well-funded attention. It could lead to healing techniques of the mind and healing technologies such as non-toxic serums, homeopathy, acupuncture and energy medicine, with profound results.

Canadian cancer researcher O. C. Gruner wrote in the early 1940s about the pleomorphists (those who recognize that microbes can change size and shape):

"The virus form, to them, is one phase in the life-history of many, if not all bacteria. The bacterial forms do not produce cancer, but the virus form does."[115]

California physicians Dr. Virginia Livingston-Wheeler and Dr. John Gregory separately treated cancer as a bacterial infection and were harassed unmercifully, despite a substantial success rate.

Dr. Gregory, because his work is less known than others, deserves some historic recognition. Al Shaefer of Florida summarizes his accomplishment as follows:

"Dr. Gregory says this microbe is as small as a virus, but not a virus. He could grow it on a non-living culture where a virus does not grow. . . .

"From the hospital where he worked Gregory obtained malignant and benign tumors and healthy tissue as determined by the pathologist. John did all his work under sterile conditions. He would grind a part of the tissue and add a portion of it to distilled water. Then he filtered this liquid through a Berkefeld filter. This sterile filter is made so that water and other objects less than the size of a micron will come through. The filter does not contaminate the liquid being filtered. It holds back all larger bacteria. John would view a tiny sample of the filtered liquid under his electron microscope. He *consistently* found the same microbe in malignant tissue. . . .

122

"Young John Gregory followed right in Koch's tracks. He isolated the microbe from malignant melanoma, cultured it, injected it into mice and baby chickens. 'Twenty-five percent of the animals developed cancers which included cancer of the ovary, adrenal, breast, stomach, spindle cell sarcoma, myosarcoma, and leukemia. A control group, ten times larger, developed no malignancies.' He isolated the microbe from the diseased animals. It was the same microbe that had been injected. It was recultured and it was the same. . . .

"John fulfilled Koch's postulates over fifty times. . . .

"But in 1964 the California Cancer Commission told John to stop using the antibiotics he developed in the treatment for the cancer-causing microbes. He was having great success. But he stopped using the antibiotics because, as his wife told us, he is a law-abiding citizen."[116]

The California Cancer Commission sounds like an official public agency. It is not. It is nine physicians of the California Medical Association, linked to the AMA, who can "outlaw" any treatment which might conflict with the financial interests of their medical union. The fact that nine men had the power to stop such a promising treatment unilaterally, with no opportunity provided for the public to influence the decision, epitomizes the central issue which this book addresses again and again—unaccountable, covert power used tyrannically, the result being the unnecessary deaths of millions.

In 1948, Dr. Virginia Livingston-Wheeler also identified the bacteria responsible for cancer. She called it *Progenitor Crytocides* (PC). Like Glover, Deaken, Gregory and others, she used a serum prepared from the individual cancer patient's urine to treat and control cancer. For legal purposes, she claims her "autogenous vaccine" treats chronic infection, but her life's work has been cancer therapy. NCI has ignored her work for decades, despite confirmation by independent researchers.

Cancer cells produce a substance called *choriogonadotropin* (CG) which coats the white blood cells and interferes with their immune function. In 1974, Dr. Livingston-Wheeler announced that her cancer microbe synthesized a CG-like material. This was confirmed by Dr. Herman Cohen and Alice Stranpp at Princeton University.[56]

Other scientists who proved the presence of and disease-causing effect of bacteria in cancer included Florence Seibert, Ph.D. and her associates at the University of Pennsylvania and later the Veterans Administration Center in Bay Pines, Florida. In her paper printed in the *New York Academy of Sciences,* Dr. Seibert described her findings and recognized the reluctance of other researchers to investigate:

"Although the presence of bacteria in tumors, surprisingly, has received attention from relatively few investigators, because they are usually assumed to be secondary invaders, logic based on pertinent results already obtained would suggest their great potential importance as possible primary invaders as well."[117]

Seibert used a density measuring apparatus to *prove pleomorphism* because the standard light microscope could not reveal the microbes in their smaller phase. Her work can be replicated by a new generation of scientists and, combined with Rife's technology, open the way to scientific acceptance of Bechamp's long-ignored work. It could also lead to the successful treatment of cancer, AIDS and other diseases.
Seibert wrote:

"The way bacteria grow into tubes of liquid media and increase in solution density (plotted curves with daily measure of the liquid culture) differs for different bacteria because of size and density in that particular medium. So when the curves of a filtrate showing nothing after filtration of that culture, but increases on daily incubation of the culture which is now clouding up and gives a curve similar to the curve of the original bacterial suspension, then we know it had gone through a pleomorphic change from visible to smaller and smaller particles until they were filterable and invisible, but on further incubation showed a typical growth curve like the original, then we knew it had transformed during its growth period. This was reported by me and others often. *Pleomorphism Proved.* (Reprints N.Y. Acad. of Sciences Annals, Vol. 141, 175, 1967; 174, 690, 1970; and Series II, 34, 506, 1972)."[118]

This certainly is too technical for the average reader to understand. It is included here to show that techniques exist which prove pleomorphism and thoroughly dispose of the argument that the bacteria discovered in laboratory tests involving cancer—such as the Memorial Sloan-Kettering test—are contaminants. They are *not* contaminants. They cause cancer and they must be addressed.

Siebert believes that a *specific* vaccine can be made from the pleomorphic (or mutant) bacteria of a specific cancer patient. That vaccine can prevent the metastasis (spread of cancer) to other parts of that specific patient's body. The vaccine should be autogenous (made from the patient's own fluids). The combination of Siebert, Rife and other pioneers offers great possibilities. The next generation of biochemists and bacteriologists would be wise to study the work and techniques of Florence Siebert.

Another interesting aspect of Siebert's work was that the pleomorphic bacteria, also called "dwarf bacteria" by some, were inhibited by DMSO. This is the molecule which caused such excitement for researchers in the mid-1960s until FDA Commissioner Goddard began persecuting it. Pat McGrady's *The Persecuted Drug: The Story of DMSO* included the following description of DMSO's effect on Siebert's pleomorphic bacteria:

> "For many years scattered scientists—mostly women—have been finding TB-type or leprosy type dwarf bacteria associated with cancer. . . . When the Siebert group added 12.5 per cent DMSO to cultures of organisms isolated from sixteen of eighteen cancer patients' tumors and blood, their growth was completely inhibited for thirty days; in control tubes there was marked growth. Siebert's discovery that the hardy, drug-defying dwarfs can be both weakened and killed by innocuous doses of DMSO encourages speculation not only that DMSO may find a place among anti-cancer drugs but also that it may lead to an anti-cancer vaccine."[22]

Pleomorphism has proved to be a key to cancer not only in the laboratory but in the clinic. Virginia Livingston-Wheeler is not the only one who has years of experience with cancer patients and good results because she recognizes pleomorphic or "dwarf" bacteria. The German cancer physician Josef Issels also had a track record of substantial success over a period of decades. His story is outlined in Appendix D at the end of this book. What is noteworthy here is that his views on the cancer

125

microbe parallel Bechamp, Rife, Gregory, Livingston-Wheeler, Seibert and others. Judith Glassman's excellent book, *The Cancer Survivors,* reported:

> "Issels thus believes that a microorganism is the immediate cause of cancer. This is the same pleomorphic microbe observed by Virginia Livingston and other researchers, growing out of the same toxic, degenerated physical condition. . . . Of this microbe, Issels says, 'Final proof has still to come because such viruses frequently assume a concealed form in cancer cells and thus cannot be readily demonstrated. Instead their presence is revealed by immunological means which detect the antigens which are the hallmark of the unseen virus.' Issels told me that he makes vaccines from antigens that cause the body to produce antibodies. 'We have here two hundred antigens. And we find out which antigen is right for each body. Then with this antigen such tumors can disappear slowly away. . . . We don't stimulate. We regenerate. If I take away the causal factors, and the secondary damage, and I change the milieu, then we make the *real* regeneration, and not just stimulation,' he told me."[54]

Milieu. Environment. Bechamp. Rife. Issels. The pieces of the solution to cancer fitting into place . . . only requiring clinics where patients have the chance to undergo such therapy—instead of the traditional burn, cut and poison.

But a new therapy demands a scientific rationale. A new biology requires theory plus laboratory proof plus clinical success. Or, to use Dr. Seibert's perceptive trinity, there is first the doer (the originating scientist or physician), followed by the viewer (who recognizes the importance of the discovery, confirms it and then promotes it), and finally the user (who applies it). Doer, Viewer, User.

John Mattingly, a pragmatic philosopher focused on the problem of integrating a new biology into today's accepted wisdom, helps us prepare for the journey ahead with these valuable compass sightings:

> "Given a speculation as to the purpose of life's cycling, we may propose that the elusive primitive living entity is a trigger cell, literally the dust of the Christian biblical story of 'from dust to dust.' If we assume the goal of medical science to be the assurance of a life span sufficiently long and free of debili-

tation to acquire maturity of spirit and consciousness, it would seem appropriate to have a very careful look at Bechamp's microzyma theory and the works of his followers. . . .

"Bechamp's original work must be translated and reviewed in a rational way; broadly seeking out convergence with recognized problems and questions in contemporary basic research in biology. The works of Bechamp's followers must also be translated and reviewed."[119]

Perhaps the slow awakening of scientists and physicians to the link between cancer and pleomorphic bacteria will finally gain momentum in the 1990s. One encouraging sign was the appearance of an article in the July 1990 issue of *Medical Hypotheses*. Dr. P. B. Macomber's "Cancer and Cell Wall Deficient Bacteria" summarized the work of the 20th century's long-ignored little band of courageous and determined researchers who defied orthodox mindset:

"Since the 1920s, a small number of researchers have been quite regularly isolating highly pleomorphic bacteria from the blood and tumors of humans and animals with cancer . . . . Only a very small number of cancer researchers today believe that bacteria play an essential role in the cancer process. Over the years, these few workers, who have carried out research supporting this concept, have generally been ignored and discredited. As a result, virtually no discussion of their work can be found in any modern textbook of oncology. Yet collectively, their research indicates that cell wall deficient bacteria are probably constantly associated with animal and human cancers . . . . This paper will attempt to outline the chief findings of these workers and propose further research to substantiate and extend their results."

In a sequel to the article on pleomorphism in *Medical Hypotheses,* Dr. Macomber addressed the profound significance of Dr. John Gregory's research (see pages 122-123). Dr. Macomber emphasized that Gregory's great contribution to understanding cancer had to be rediscovered. Modern researchers simply had to reconstruct Gregory's work, using today's technology and knowledge. Macomber wrote in "Cancer and Cell Wall Deficient Bacteria Part II" (unpublished at the time this update was going to press):

"Gregory concluded that essentially all human cancers (and

presumably all cancers) contain *living viral particles* which are an *essential* component of these cancers and which appear responsible for the fundamental nature of cancer.

"Gregory has demonstrated that cancer 'viruses' . . . are, by the strict biological definition of viruses, really small bacteria since they can grow on lifeless media and do not absolutely require living cells for their growth . . .

"He discoverd an antibiotic from a strain of Rhizopus which he named 'antivin' . . . He found that cancer cells but not their cancer viruses were destroyed by therapy with X-ray and alkylating agents. In contrast, tumor tissue from patients treated with antivin, showed destruction of both cancer cells and viruses . . .

"With the antigenic nature of the viruses readily available for study, it may be possible to develop very effective vaccines which could completely protect both humans and their animal food sources . . . against most cancer viruses.

"In summary, Dr. John E. Gregory deserves nomination for the title of "the Robert Koch of cancer.' Once his work has been confirmed and brought up to date by modern research techniques, he will have proven beyond any reasonable doubt that cancer viruses . . . are the essential cause of all cancers . . . Any scientist . . . can begin confirming and extending his findings. The bulk of modern cancer research and therapy has apparently been misdirected at studying and trying to remove or destroy the cancer cell rather than the cancer viruses which are responsible for the 'antisocial behavior' of the cancer cell. We must now rapidly redirect research and therapeutic efforts toward cancer viruses."

Chapter Ten

# Three Davids vs. The Goliaths

*"The hero's main feat is to overcome the monster of darkness."*

Carl Jung

The world changes because men and women make it change. Orthodox medicine and "big science" are powerful but not all-powerful. They do play dirty. Yet against this darkness are shafts of light—individuals and organizations who by their solitary efforts give hope to those who are trapped in the nightmare. Three examples are provided here—three Davids who have stood against the Goliaths and who have lit the way for other men and women to follow.

## DAVID #1

Walter Nelson-Rees managed the best cell bank in the United States in Oakland, California. In the 1970s, he began exposing the fact that numerous cancer cell lines used in research were contaminated by the infamous HeLa cell. Cell lines from Russia, Germany, China and numerous other nations were contaminated by a particularly aggressive HeLa cell from a Baltimore, Maryland woman who died in 1951. For example, researchers who thought they were experimenting with male prostate cancer cells were in fact using female glandular cells. Over one-third of the cancer cell lines used for research were contaminated. Monkey viruses began appearing in human cells as a result of the mix-up. A potential nightmare for cancer research existed.

Nelson-Rees tried to warn scientists through an article in *Science*. But the editor contemptuously rejected the article until Nelson-Rees found backing at NCI. Then it was published and a storm broke (1974).

However, business as usual continued. The NCI published research on lung cancer in April 1977 but took a year to publish Nelson-Rees' criticism that the earlier research was worthless because of cell line contamination. Scientists wasted a year following the false trail because NCI officials didn't want to "rock the boat."

Nelson-Rees was considered the guardian of pure cell lines by the honest researchers. But the ones whose work was revealed to be worthless by Nelson-Rees were out to get him. In 1980, the opposition was strong enough to go after him. NCI decided to cut the small budget ($600,000) of perhaps the most critical cell bank in the world. In 1981, they permanently closed the facility. The reason: budgetary constraints. Yet they spend *one and a half billion dollars a year* on white elephant research, travel, grants to the favored, rigged evaluations of successful clinics such as Burton's, etc., etc., etc. As Nelson-Rees wailed when the NCI chiefs brought out their knives:

> "Do they actually have to be told why it was necessary to safeguard the most widely used experimental material in cancer research?"[93]

NCI's budget was $958 million a year when they decided to close the Walter Nelson-Rees cell bank because of "budgetary cutbacks." NCI's billion and a half dollar budget of today ignores the matter of keeping cell lines pure.

The American Cancer Society grabs perhaps $400 million a year from the American public. Historically its research budget has been less than 30% of what it collects from millions of uninformed Americans. No major cancer breakthrough in treatment has ever resulted from an ACS grant recipient.

Memorial Sloan-Kettering reportedly receives $70 million a year from tax-exempt foundations and tax-deductible personal contributions. Its fees for treatment bring in much more. It staunchly defends chemotherapy, radiation and surgery.

The University of Texas Cancer Center had a budget of $250 million in fiscal year 1984-85.

Yet $600,000 is too much to preserve the purity of the cell lines for cancer research!

Of course money was not the real reason the cell bank was closed. Nelson-Rees had exposed the work of some top members of "the old boy network" as absolutely worthless. They went after him. They got him. But he stood at conventions and denounced them. He refused to be political and "go along" even though his friends advised him to do so. He told the truth. History will appreciate him. And someday, somewhere, perhaps a new cell bank will come into existence. Its standards will be of the highest . . . and Walter Nelson-Rees will be remembered.

## DAVID #2

Ralph Auer came out of the conservative midwestern soil of Indiana. He graduated from West Point and was commissioned an officer in the United States Army. He served in the Korean War, taking a submachine gun slug through his right wrist and into his chest, leaving the right side of his right hand paralyzed. Later he became an aerospace engineer and then a manufacturer's representative for medical electronic equipment and devices. He was a solid, patriotic American citizen who believed in the system. Then his wife developed breast cancer in 1979.

The orthodox medical men put her on the treadmill—surgery, radiation, chemotherapy, surgery, more surgery, more radiation, more chemotherapy. Finally Ralph Auer began looking into alternative therapies in Mexico, the Bahamas and elsewhere. Slowly he read the medical literature and learned what his wife had been denied until it was too late. Ralph Auer's wife died on January 31, 1988. Nine years of struggling with breast cancer were over. Since she had lived five years, she went into the official statistics as "cured."

On November 1, 1988 Ralph Auer paid for an ad in his local newspaper, the *Carmel Valley Sun* in California. The ad was his way of informing others who had cancer of the facts he had learned through the years. It was the act of a solitary citizen standing up and denouncing the American Cancer Society and the National Cancer Institute for their lies and supression of alternative therapies.

After quoting from a number of professional articles which contradicted the official views, Ralph Auer listed the names of alternative cancer organizations. Then he concluded with these words:

> "Or you can simply contact me whether you would like more information or would like for me to talk to you and a group of your friends. I care."

The phone began ringing. People—average citizens like Ralph Auer—called to thank him, ask him for more information, and encourage him in his fight with the giant cancer organizations. Then the director of the local American Cancer Society called. She asked if Mr. Auer would be willing to meet with the President of the California branch of the American Cancer Society. The ACS obviously was upset with the ad and wanted to see if they could placate Ralph Auer.

It was, of course, the American Cancer Society and the Cancer Commission of the California Medical Association who had made it impossible for Ralph Auer's wife to receive the alternative therapy of her choice.

> "In 1966 the ACS formulated a State Model Cancer Act which was instrumental in the enactment of anti-quackery laws now enforced in 9 states. . . . In California, (it is a) . . . felony . . .
>
> "The use of unproven methods is also a criminal offense in Colorado, Illinois, Kentucky, Maryland, Nevada, North Dakota, Ohio and Pennsylvania." [120]

New York is the same. As Patrick McGrady Jr. reminds us:

> "The definition of malpractice in New York state, as it is in many other states in this country, is to operate outside the mainstream of medical oncology. You can be convicted. You can be fined. You can lose your license. You can go to jail. People can bring malpractice suits against you even if releases have been signed.
>
> "It is now illegal to find a cure for cancer."[26]

Nevertheless, Ralph Auer decided to meet the enemy—the American Cancer Society. He invited this author to accompany him.

Ralph Auer and Dr. Lowell Irwin, President of the California division of the American Cancer Society met on November 4, 1988 in Salinas, California (where John Steinbeck immortalized the struggle of those on the bottom against those on the top).

Auer asked Dr. Irwin if he agreed with the ACS statement of March 5, 1987 that, "Caught early enough, breast cancer has cure rates approaching 100 percent." Dr. Irwin stated he totally agreed with the statement. And so the exchange began.

It soon became apparent to this author that Dr. Irwin was not interested in an honest discussion of the issues. He gave long-winded speeches about his medical career and concern for his patients. He tried to emphasize the good done by the ACS educational program, particularly the anti-smoking campaign. He totally ignored the ACS's unwillingness to fight the tobacco lobby where it counted—in the pits in Washington, D.C. As Peter Barry Chowka showed in his 1978 exposure of the ACS, their anti-tobacco activities were safe and self-serving:

> "ACS' identification with the anti-smoking campaign is largely public relations posturing. . . . Considerable evidence exists to implicate a variety of environmental factors . . . in the twentieth century lung cancer epidemic."[37]

Dr. Irwin refused to discuss substance. He claimed to know little or nothing of the work of people such as Dr. Burzynski of Houston who was on the ACS quack list. Yet Dr. Irwin was a cancer specialist.

Again and again, Dr. Irwin fell back on statistics to justify ACS positions, but the statistics were questionable. When statistics were brought forth by Ralph Auer which were detrimental to ACS' positions, such as Dr. Bailar's devastating May 1986 *New England Journal of Medicine* article, Dr. Irwin simply dismissed Bailar with the wave of a hand. The issue of suppression of legitimate cures originated by men and women on the ACS "hit" list also was not a subject open for discussion. The question of conspiracy was not seriously tackled. "Do you believe there is a conspiracy" asked Dr. Irwin near the end of the one hour meeting. Ralph Auer responded by quoting the U.S. Senate report of Ben Fitzgerald:

"My investigation to date should convince this committee that a conspiracy does exist."

Ralph Auer unswervingly refused to budge from his position despite an hour of Dr. Irwin's patronizing putdowns.

Irwin had the opportunity to learn a great deal from a man who saw the ACS and cancer procedures from a totally different perspective. But Irwin wasn't interested. I concluded that Irwin was intellectually dishonest. His job was to defend the ACS, enjoy the glitter of the fund-raising activities, and, if called upon, try to seductively silence the occasional outraged citizen such as Ralph Auer. Auer was a potential nightmare for the fund-raising efforts of that ACS chapter, the second most successful in all of California.

But with Auer, Dr. Irwin failed miserably. Auer wasn't simply a bereaved husband who could be quieted by a smiling politician with "Doctor" in front of his name who insisted on emphasizing the "Mister" when he addressed Ralph Auer. Auer was a West Point trained combat veteran who, like millions of other Americans, had served his country in war because be believed in American freedom. Auer was also an engineer, entrepreneur and student of the medical literature. He was the ACS' worst nightmare—the educated, enraged citizen who recognized the ACS racket.

When Ralph Auer is joined by others, and citizens start forming alternative organizations to the ACS, and the media and Congress finally start paying attention to how the average citizen is being tortured and murdered by orthodox cancer treatment, then perhaps the solitary act of Ralph Auer will be seen in a light similar to the defiant act of Rosa Parks who refused to move to the back of a bus in 1955, and thus started the Civil Rights Movement of the 1960s.

Ralph Auer's provocative and courageous advertisement from the November 1, 1988 *Carmel Valley Sun* is reproduced in its entirety at the end of this book as Appendix A. Selections from Ben Fitzgerald's Senate investigation report into the cancer establishment are included as Appendix B.

Following Ralph Auer's meeting with the President of the California ACS, Auer placed another newspaper advertisement in the *Monterey Herald*. One irate reader responded with a letter to the editor which stated that "to condemn the good work of the American Cancer Society . . . should not be tolerated."

Not be tolerated? What did that mean? Not allowed to be printed? Censorship? The writer was Richard B. Levine of Monterey, seemingly just a citizen who disagreed with Ralph Auer. Or was he? Auer did a little checking and soon discovered that Levine was Dr. Levine. Doctor Levine was masquerading as merely a private citizen having no vested interest in the matter. Dr. Levine was a radiologist and member of the local medical society. Dishonesty and misleading the public on such a basic point, as well as arguing the position that open, free discussion of the cancer alternatives and criticism of the establishment "should not be tolerated" (despite the Constitution's guarantee of free speech) should make every citizen pause. Pause and thank Ralph Auer for flushing out such views from one of the "Gods in White Coats."

## DAVID #3

Dr. Dick Richards was a private physician working in England. He turned away from orthodox treatment for cancer patients after witnessing its horrible effects. He found that the "Gentle Method" produced far better results, even when the patient died. His "Gentle Method" was premised on letting the body's own regenerative ability come forth by providing appropriate help, rather than immune-suppressing poisons. He wrote:

> "Using the Gentle Method nearly always produces an early response in the patient. There is usually a rapid decrease in pain and a progressive feeling of improvement in a number of ways."[13]

The Gentle Method consisted of a variety of alternative approaches. There was no rigid procedure, but rather a personal program based on the patient's condition. The patient and the patient's family were critically important. Diet and psychological attitude played important roles. Daily treatment of the body was emphasized, either with the physician's help, as with injections or without the physician, as with diet.

135

Among the modalities used by Dr. Richards, when appropriate, was BCG, a weakened strain of the tuberculosis bacteria—in order to stimulate the immune system. Other therapies included enemas, mega-vitamins, minerals and laetrile. Laetrile was "markedly helpful"—no cure-all, no dramatic effect, but "markedly helpful" in an appropriate situation. His number one rule was that "there should be no further harm done to the patient."

He converted from orthodox treatment when a patient of his, a schoolteacher, pleaded with him to try something different after the patient had undergone surgery for lung cancer, months of chemotherapy, and had only three to four weeks to live. Dr. Richard's own words convey the significance of the Gentle Method:

> "He died. But he died eleven months later. And what a difference while he lived. Not only did he actually return to school for over a term, but he played golf, enjoyed his family, and grew an entire extra year's crop in his garden . . . something he declared to be the biggest bonus of all. He was active and happy until ten days before his death. I was converted. I believe that other doctors trying this method on one or two such late cases would be converted, too."[13]

Dr. Richards no longer practices in England. But his "Gentle Method" and his 1982 book *The Topic of Cancer* helped show the way. As the influential London Times editorialized on June 26, 1990:

> "The British Medical Association has acknowledged at last that alternative medicine is not quackery . . . The boom in alternative medicine has occurred independent of the state and of most of the profession, a triumph for the free market . . . Encouraging results have been achieved by the—still cautious—use of holistic therapies in treatment for cancer at the Hammersmith Hospital . . .
>
> "A profession whose greatest experts could deceive themselves for so long should encompass novelty with humility."

## Chapter Eleven

# The Answer to Cancer

*"It is now illegal to find a cure for cancer."*
Pat McGrady Jr.[26]

*"Remember, remember always that all of us, and you and I especially, are descended from immigrants and revolutionists."*
President Franklin Roosevelt

The answer to cancer can come only through fundamental changes in the structure of medicine and the regulations regarding treatment. Without a determined movement by people who understand the issues, no changes are possible on a national scale. For the immediate future, state legislatures and even city councils must be the battleground. And until one state or city courageously offers alternative treatments, protected from AMA medical boards and FDA invasions, cancer cures will be available only to the wealthy who can travel outside the United States. It is undemocratic for the vast majority of the public to be denied treatment that works while the wealthy or the few who are informed are healed of cancer.

It is certain that any state or city which attempts to set up an alternative treatment facility will be put under enormous pressure by the medical establishment, drug companies and perhaps even criminals specializing in intimidation to halt any reform attempts. But a few states already have homeopathic medical boards separate from the allopathic AMA boards (Arizona, Nevada and Connecticut). Other states allow bio-electronic treatment on a small scale. The treatment of cancer by such devices should be legislated.

It is important to keep in mind that labor unions won their

right to exist in the 1930s because the state of Michigan and its courageous governor faced down the goons hired by the Ford Motor Company. Labor unions need to recognize they are confronting a similar enemy in the Medical Monopoly, and that their members' lives are at risk. Labor unions could be an essential ally in an alternative cancer therapy movement. As a group, labor unions are now closely wedded to the Medical Monopoly through their health programs, but individual chapters are where calls for a radical change in cancer treatment could emerge. This is particularly true in industries where cancer and other untreatable diseases are widespread among union workers.

Successful business leaders constitute another group where isolated support for alternative cancer therapies might be found. If only a few business leaders of national prominence would cross the line and endorse publicly an alternative cancer approach, it could have a significant impact. While business executives tend to be politically conservative, many of the brightest men and women at the higher levels are particularly well-educated and free-thinking. Some certainly are mavericks and any corrupt, incompetent and dangerous monopoly, particularly one that threatens the health of their families and employees, could quickly become the target of their considerable skills. It would require only a few such business executives to start a mass awakening followed by mass outrage at what has been and is being done to American citizens. If nothing else, the participation of a number of business executives in helping to finance a new private cancer organization dedicated to educating the public and testing alternatives would be helpful. If such associations should be blocked because of pressure or illegal acts, then we truly have lost our Constitutional Rights.

It is essential that alternative treatments be tested objectively and be well-documented. The highest scientific standards need to be applied in order to evaluate these therapies which have been kept so long from the American public.

And yet, given the 10,000 Americans who die of cancer every week, there ought to be a recognized right for all patients, giving them the freedom to choose therapies they believe might help them. On April 30, 1987, the U.S. Court of Appeals for the Second Circuit ruled that each citizen did have such a right. The case involved Dr. Emanuel Revici of New York, a pioneer whose alternative approaches and successful treatments had infuriated the orthodox authorities. Operating in the heart of the beast—New York—Revici has been one of the Medical Monopoly's prime targets for years. The victory by Revici and his patients caused earthquake tremors under the legal foundation of the cancer profiteers. A Supreme Court decision upholding the right of patients to choose their own therapies would give all American citizens the option of alternative treatment.

The U.S. Federal Court of Appeals for New York ruled:

"We see no reason why a patient should not be allowed to make an informed decision to go outside currently approved medical methods in search of an unconventional treatment. . . . An informed decision to avoid surgery and chemotherapy is within the patient's right to determine what to do with his or her own body."

It is unlikely that the U.S. Justice Department will do its duty and initiate a full investigation of the criminal conspiracy, monopolistic practices, anti-trust actions and murderous results of the FDA-AMA-NCI-ACS syndicate. But a courageous law firm, motivated by an heroic impulse, could bring a massive class action suit. Many families who have lost members could be the aggrieved parties. Such a private legal initiative is long overdue, and every day that it doesn't happen reveals to the world how we, as citizens of the oldest democracy in the world, have apparently lost our nerve and consequently our freedom.

A teacher of mine once told me that the fight for freedom must be constantly waged. As a college student I did not understand. I naïvely thought Americans had won most of their freedoms. Economic rights were still to be achieved, but no other huge "right" to be gained was visible on my horizon. How wrong I was and how poorly I knew my nation's history at that time.

It was one of our founding fathers who began the struggle

for Medical Freedom. Dr. Benjamin Rush, an original signer of the Declaration of Independence, fought for this right at the very beginning of the great American experiment. As with the abolition of slavery, the women's vote and other neglected rights, Medical Freedom was not granted at the nation's inception. They all had to wait until their time—when an overwhelming public thrust or national crisis forced the political leaders to rectify a grievous wrong. Dr. Raymond Keith Brown, whose recommendations for changing the FDA were quoted earlier, wrote the following about Dr. Benjamin Rush:

> "That well-known physician of the Colonial era, and signer of the Declaration of Independence, opposed official recognition of any one system of medicine, much as the Constitution forbade the establishment of a state religion."[25]

Despite the efforts of corrupt government officials, a monopolistic doctor's trust and a fraudulent American Cancer Society, Dr. Rush's words are as alive and relevant today as when they were uttered over 200 years ago:

> "Unless we put Medical Freedom into the Constitution, the time will come when medicine will organize into an undercover dictatorship. To restrict the art of healing to one class of men and deny equal privileges to others will constitute the Bastille of medical science. All such laws are un-American and despotic. They are fragments of monarchy and have no place in a republic. The Constitution of this Republic should make special provisions for Medical Freedom as well as Religion Freedom."

Dr. Bruce Halstead, who suffered by opposing the Medical Monopoly, described how California law prevents a dedicated physician from honoring the Hippocratic Oath:

> "The present laws under Title 21, Food, Drug and Cosmetic Act, and California Health and Safety Code Section 1707.1, prohibit a physician or anyone else from prescribing a food product, compound, or a device used in nutritional support of a cancer patient or a patient suffering from any other disease. Any time a food product is related to a disease process, the food automatically becomes an 'unapproved drug.'

> "The cancer patient is not only a victim of the disease, but the victim of a diabolical system which dictates that once

surgery, radiation and chemotherapy have failed, it is illegal for a physician to provide the cancer victim any nutritional support, even if it is given to them gratis. This is the law in the state of California."[121]

The laws are similar in other states. Dr. Thomas Roberts of Virginia lost his medical license when he included nutritional supplements for his cancer patients. The Medical Boards in every state relentlessly enforce the anti-food policy of Morris Fishbein, who never practiced medicine a day in his life but fundamentally corrupted the health system of the United States for almost the entire 20th century.

The need for a Medical Freedom right is essential.

> "I do not think it is the job of the government to protect people from themselves. I do think it is legitimate for the FDA . . . to help educate the public. That is part of their mandate. . . . But having said that, the government should be only one of the competing voices in terms of educating the public."
>
> Dr. Franz Engelfinder,
> former editor of
> *The New England Journal of Medicine*

> "Nobody has full knowledge. To say that FDA has full knowledge and you poor people out there are ignorant . . . is ridiculous."
>
> Dr. Michael J. Halberstam, commenting on
> FDA Commissioner Kennedy's claim that
> Medical Freedom couldn't be given to the
> public because they didn't have
> "full knowledge."[52]

When Medical Freedom is finally established as a legal right, with all the difficult new problems it will inevitably bring as hucksters try to cash in, at least it will enable conscientious physicians and researchers to establish, through objective methods, whether dozens of existing, inexpensive therapies offer a desperate patient the chance for real healing. If such a change happens, one group that will deserve the appreciation of the nation will be the gays. Most fair-minded Americans recognize that it is the gays, because of AIDS, who have helped cause an enormous crack in the Medical Monopoly's wall. Gays made the FDA cancer and AIDS politics obvious to millions. The state of California even opened its own agency to approve potentially useful, non-FDA approved drugs for patients with AIDS. The New York Circuit Court ruling on Medical Freedom, combined with California's approval system for new drugs, offer models to other states to go even further.

In July 1988, a newly formed "Physicians Association for AIDS Care," a national association based in Oakbrook Terrace, Illinois, began organizing to serve as an alternative to the big health centers where most new drugs are clinically tested. The group has 300 members and will enable new drugs to reach patients outside the medical centers. While the group is closely tied to the drug companies and for that reason is unlikely to bring about revolutionary healing, its existence demonstrates how decentralization is the only viable alternative to the rigid national health conspiracy which now exists. With new state laws, and many alternative therapies available, Medical Freedom could be a practical reality in a few years time.

If that happens, then the day could come when the heterosexual men of America witness their parent, wife or child saved from a deadly cancer because the gays' combativeness helped change the system. The whole nation could owe the gays an enormous debt of gratitude.

Another group of people who deserve the nation's thanks are those who practiced and developed the "unproven" therapies. This includes physicians who quietly oppose the orthodox ways and utilize futuristic methods when appropriate. It includes physicians forced to practice in Mexico, the Bahamas or elsewhere in order to provide techniques or substances which are "unapproved." It includes non-physicians who have learned or discovered procedures which produce results, although official medicine won't examine them objectively. It includes bio-electronic healers who heal serious diseases and never tell the patients how sick they truly are—just making them well in a month or two when orthodox ways would put them in their graves. It includes outlaw physicians who give workshops and move from place to place, one step ahead of medical officials and ambitious district attorneys. It includes spiritual healers who work with energies that are dismissed by the purely materialistic scientists—even though advanced physicists have long since proved such rigid, purely materialistic views of the universe to be utter, absolute nonsense and second-rate science.

Research institutions which openly test and evaluate this spectrum of procedures are long overdue. But because of the cancer conspiracy, no such pioneering places can operate openly or can announce the results publicly. It is amusing that a Vice-President of Memorial Sloan-Kettering admitted to Ralph Moss that the ACS "hit" list was "where they got all their best ideas." [26]

In other words, stomp on the innovator but steal his or her discoveries and legitimize them for profit at Memorial Sloan-Kettering. There's a word for such activities—the word is "racketeering."

One of the devices used by the Medical Monopoly to thwart testing of alternative therapies is the demand for double-blind studies, involving a group which receives a placebo. Many, many physicians recognize that double-blind testing is phony. Yet, because of the expenses and organizational demands, the double-blind criterion is a convenient tool to keep alternative therapies from being fairly evaluated. Most doctors realize that "historic controls" are simpler, equally valid from a scientific perspective, and not as ethically questionable: in a double-blind study those receiving the placebo are being duped while their lives hang in the balance.

"Historical controls" simply means assessing the group being provided with the experimental therapy against similar groups using traditional therapy. It certainly can be used in the first phase of an experimental trial. It cuts down on costs and speeds up the process of bringing new therapies to the hospital beds.

Naturally the "scientists" at NCI and ACS detest the notion of historical controls. But then, their interests have been shown to be different from those of the patients, haven't they? It is the *separation* of scientific inquiry and the process of identifying effective new therapies which is the issue crying for attention. Years of abusing the patient and the individual

143

physician are what has resulted from all the control and authorizing procedures being handed over to the NCI-FDA types.

"Historical controls" were described simply and precisely as follows by *Toronto Star* reporter Lillian Newberry:

"Dr. Agnes Klein of the bureau of human prescription drugs in Ottawa says . . . the key consideration in any study is that it does not jeopardize patients . . .

". . . use 'historical controls' as a comparison group when you have an illness that invariably results in death no matter what the current treatment, she says. You give a group of patients the proposed new treatment and compare their outcome with the medical records of a matched group who had the disease."[122]

"Historical controls" are an obvious keystone of any extensive alternative therapy legislated by a state or city willing to make history for Medical Freedom. In truth, historical controls are the *primary* way of medical advancement. Dr. Larry Siegel of Key West, Florida has declared:

"I can't think of a single major medical advance that occurred in an atmosphere of double-blind placebo control studies with the clear support of the medical establishment behind it. . . . Every advance has occurred with someone with some decent thinking behind their work trying something new."[123]

There is also the recognized medical tradition that "dramatic therapeutic effects," especially with conditions which invariably lead to death, can eliminate not only the need for double-blind trials but even the historical controls comparison. The NCI, FDA and other gatekeepers simply won't permit the "dramatic therapeutic effects"—a medical tradition—to be recognized in cancer treatment. The thousands of documented case histories of both Hoxsey and Ivy (Krebiozen), which demonstrated antitumor activity and which were rejected by NCI and FDA officials, attest to the reluctance of the authorities to recognize anything outside their controlled approach.

In discussing this important element of any future alternative cancer evaluation, Robert G. Houston has written:

"Leading experts on cancer clinical trials, such as Freireich

(1975) and Carter (1985) have pointed out that dramatic therapeutic effects obviate the need for controlled trials of effectiveness."[48]

Patrick McGrady, Jr. adds:

"If you have a biological treatment that really creates a good response in human cancer patients you know this without comparing them. What a randomized control trial does—and there are places for them in oncology—it shows you fine differences, but you don't need it for a breakthrough."[26]

As for safety, only *short-term* safety can be determined anyhow—in any clinical trial. As Walter S. Ross made clear in his 1977 book, *The Life/Death Ratio:*

"Clinical testing can detect only short-term, frequent adverse reactions. Nobody can tell what the long-term, infrequent side effects of drugs will be until they have been taken for years or decades by large numbers of people."

When the issue is *terminal cancer,* the super-cautious, bureaucratic procedure now in existence, further restricted by demands for expensive double-blind studies requiring months or years to prepare and directed only by highly credentialed experts, all approved by orthodox committees, is not only absurd, it is criminal.

The point being argued here—and it is critical—is that double-blind tests often are used as a clever technique to keep promising alternative therapies from being tried or evaluated. Once a new method appears to be successful when compared with "historical controls," *then* it is important to use double-blind tests to ensure its effectiveness and safety—before it is widely used. But using the double-blind criteria as a way to keep the innovative therapies from being tested needs to be recognized as the orthodox-status quo medicine trick that it is. The following two quotations present both sides of a difficult issue.

From "Institutionalized Ignorance" by Alan R. Gaby, M.D., published in *The Townsend Letter for Doctors,* December 1988:

"The average physician is afraid to be the first to try something new. He or she therefore depends on the opinions of so-called 'experts' or 'authorities,' who write review articles in medical journals. The problem is that these individuals are usually experts not in the area they are evaluating, but in the conventional methods that directly compete with the new therapy."[124]

Dr. Bernard Fisher, noted breast cancer and clinical trials expert, was quoted in *Target: Cancer* by Edward J. Sylvester as follows:

> "The introduction of prospective randomized clinical trials into clinical medicine would surely make order out of chaos. . . . When properly employed such trials could undoubtedly provide definitive information relative to the worth of therapies prior to their widespread use on populations as a whole . . ."[8]

One further point needs to be emphasized. There is substantial evidence that orthodox medicine uses *rigged* double-blind studies when it wishes to discredit a therapy it opposes. Nobel Prize winner Linus Pauling claims that this is exactly what happened with the Vitamin C trials at the Mayo Clinic in Minnesota. Earlier trials by Ewan Cameron, M.D. in Scotland showed terminal cancer patients lived *four times longer* with improved quality of life when administered large doses of Vitamin C. A Japanese trial produced similar results. Then the Mayo Clinic did two trials with Vitamin C and claimed the earlier trials were wrong. Pauling protested, pointing out (correctly) that the Mayo tests weren't the same. They included chemotherapy as well as Vitamin C! Yet the orthodox experts still point to the Mayo trials as disproving the Vitamin C claims. This is scientific dishonesty at its most blatant. To have it come from such a respected institution as the Mayo Clinic shows how extensive the corruption in the cancer world has become.

There is also little doubt that NCI rigged the national laetrile studies in the mid-70s and then again in the early 80s. The mid-70s rigging is the most interesting and obvious. Dean Burk, Ph.D. was head of the Department of Cell Chemistry at the NCI for 34 years. When NCI "tested" laetrile in 1973 and reported it had failed, Burk blew the whistle. He described to interested Congressmen how the tests had showed exactly the opposite result—laetrile had been proven effective. In a letter to Congressman Robert A. Roe, Dr. Burk explained why the cancer hierarchy had to cover up laetrile's effectiveness:

> "Once any of the FDA-NCI-AMA-ACS hierarchy so much as concede that laetrile antitumor efficacy was indeed once observed in NCI experimentation, a permanent crack in the bureaucratic armor has taken place that can widen indefinitely by further appropriate experimentation."[125]

Later that year, NCI conducted a massive test of laetrile at an independent research institute. Again the government announced that laetrile was worthless. *The trial was a total fraud*.

Years later, a fellow of the Royal Statistical Society in London told me that any amateur statistician could see the flaws. Apparently that was what the American medical and scientific communities wanted, he concluded. The interest in laetrile eventually faded. The cover-up succeeded.

The statistical expert stated that there was "one chance in four billion that those results which were positive for laetrile could have occurred by chance." Details of this fraudulent trial can be found in Appendix E. The point to keep in mind is that while laetrile is not effective against tumors, some ingredient in the "apricot kernal soup" is exceptionally effective. But no scientists are interested in finding out what it is. The politics is the issue, not the science. Meanwhile, millions die because of such monstrous infamy.

The public realizes that something is terribly wrong—that organized scientific dishonesty operates often, particularly when powerful vested interests are threatened. But with no governmental leadership opposing such covert activities, rampant media cowardice, and the absence of any noteworthy grass roots leadership fighting for Medical Freedom, the public's discontent can only be registered through public opinion polls, when the dissatisfaction starts to bubble up from below:

> "A surprising national poll by Associated Press/Media General found that more than half of the American public feels so-called unorthodox cancer clinics should be allowed to operate freely in the United States. Because there is a virtual media

blackout on potentially positive information about alternative cancer treatments, this sentiment indicates a profoundly grass roots movement probably stemming from direct personal experience. This is the first time since the '50s that such signs have been present."[32]

In December 1985, NCI began promoting Interleukin-2, developed by Steven A. Rosenberg, M.D., Chief of Surgery at the National Cancer Institute. They claimed a 44% reduction in cancer tumors in previously untreatable cases. Dr. Robert Oldham, an NCI renegade, opened a private clinic and began using Interleukin-2 for wealthy patients who were charged as much as $35,000 for the treatment. Over 1000 physicians were referring patients to Dr. Oldham, according to his press statements. Yet, three years later, the miracle Interleukin-2 was reported to be effective in not 44%, but only 30%, and more important, the tumor shrinkage was temporary. In addition, Interleukin-2, like the earlier fiasco Interferon, was highly toxic. After a few patients died because of it, NCI pulled back on its propaganda.[126]

The one positive result that comes from Dr. Oldham's "alternative treatment" is that despite opposition from NCI, ACS and the FDA, he and his company have been permitted to continue because there is a loophole. Lawrence Surtees, a reporter for the Toronto *Globe and Mail,* explained:

> "The U.S. Food and Drug Administration has allowed only six centres, sponsored by the NCI, to conduct trials of the experimental treatment. However, FDA rules allow doctors to provide experimental treatments to consenting patients on a last resort basis, and this is what the company is doing."[127]

Given this allowance, the fact of the public's discontent, and the "Medical Freedom" call from the grave by one of the signers of the Declaration of Independence, it is certainly an acceptable position for a new generation of political leaders to begin introducing numerous Medical Freedom statutes in city council halls, state legislatures and even in the national Congress. Even if Medical Freedom were initially restricted to a clinic where a qualified M.D., homeopathic physician or chiropractor were in charge, it would enable many of the new therapeutic approaches to be used for consenting citizens who wanted them. Alternative therapists, acupuncturists and energy medicine practitioners could easily operate under such an arrangement—at least in the beginning, until various therapies had developed sufficient documentation for objective evaluation.

As the situation stands now, only the NCI, FDA, AMA and ACS, with their various affiliated medical centers, *dictate* treatment. With the cover-ups, political influence and outright suppression that have been shown to exist, such monopolistic tyranny for the sake of scientism should not remain unchallenged. Citizens need to protest, petition their representatives, form state associations, pester their media and holler until "Medical Freedom" bills start appearing in City Council chambers and state legislatures. Then perhaps the national Congress will rediscover what democracy is about and challenge the monster.

The British statesman Benjamin Disraeli once said, "The health of the people is really the foundation upon which all their happiness and all their powers as a state depend." Politicians who won't face the truths presented in this book, and who are unwilling to take a position on "Medical Freedom" because they fear the power of the AMA-FDA-NCI-ACS syndicate, must be replaced. They have no comprehension of their fundamental duties as elected representatives and lawmakers in a democratic society.

But new laws are only one necessary element of what must be done. Equally serious is the recognition that medical experts of all kinds, if they are to be allowed to continue to keep any authority, must be responsible to a higher authority—democratic judgment. General Dwight Eisenhower, leading the Allied invasion of Europe in World War II, recognized that an army of a democracy needed to be informed—the soldiers had to understand what and why they were fighting. The medical generals must be held accountable also, in ways appropriate to the democratic society which they serve.

Paul Feyerabend, a university scholar, has described the problem and the solution:

> "Laymen can and must supervise science. It would not only
> be foolish but downright irrresponsible to accept the judgment

149

of scientists . . . without further examination. If the matter is important, either to a small group or to society as a whole, then this judgment must be subjected to the most painstaking scrutiny. . . . Duly elected committees of laymen must examine. . . . That the errors of specialists can be discovered by ordinary people, provided they are prepared to do some hard work, is the basic assumption of any trial by jury. The law demands that experts be cross-examined . . . science is not beyond the reach of the natural shrewdness of the human race. I suggest that this shrewdness be applied to all important social matters which are now in the hands of experts."[128]

This issue is critical—democractic supervision. Doctors and hospital administrators are adamantly opposed to it. But it is a principle which in time could and should become deeply rooted in the planet's social evolution. Just as almost everyone in America accepts the wisdom that civilian control over the military is absolutely essential for the survival of democratic values and institutions, so the civilian control over the doctors has an equally compelling rationale.

As for the issue of a civilian "jury" being able to make wise decisions, Feyerabend is not the only person who has thought about the issue and decided in favor of the community and the average citizen. Washington Post columnist Charles Krauthammer wrote in late 1988:

"Biology is very complicated, but in principle it is comprehensible. Give a jury of your peers an hour and they can gain a reasonable grasp of, say, immunology."

As for how local communities select their supervising juries, that is a local decision and may call for different formulas in different locations.

The spectacle of local community groups overseeing cancer therapies and demanding communication and answers from those who treat cancer and AIDS patients may be difficult for the reader to accept. There exists the possibility of abuses and local corruption. But the national program has already been exposed as inherently corrupt and abusive to the public. With so much power and money controlling these institutions, reform is not possible. So the decentralized, local solution is mandatory. Combined with the patients' self-interest and responsibility in choosing the alternative therapy option, local and state control over cancer therapy is the obvious answer. In the case of corrupt, incompetent or intimidated local officials, the citizen has the option of going elsewhere. When viewed against the outrageous fees and expenses needed to travel out of the country now to Mexican or European clinics, the option of traveling to another state, or a different community within a state, is a simple and obvious alternative. What awaits the cancer patient under the existing Medical Monopoly is almost certain death.

As Maryann Napol has written:

"Radiation and chemotherapy—either separately or in combination—are generally used as adjuncts to cancer surgery. Each is a double-edged sword: surgery may be responsible for the spread of cancer, according to many physicians; radiation is itself a carcinogen (cancer-causing agent); anticancer drugs are highly toxic and, in many cases, carcinogenic."[42]

Dr. George Crile, Jr., Emeritus Surgeon of the Cleveland Clinic, once noted:

"Biopsies . . . should be undertaken with the greatest caution. . . . Even needle biopsy does not appear to be safe. . . . It gives credence to what our patients already think and tell us—that cutting into cancer spreads it and makes it grow.[7]

Doctor William D. Kelley supported this view and exposed the deception at the heart of the biopsy process. The search for truth among cancer specialists was abandoned so long ago that few question the money-making assumptions (such as biopsies, chemotherapy, etc.) any longer. Dr. Kelley:

"Biopsy tells nothing of other tumors or other metastases in the body at the same time. Many times the physician will take a biopsy of a breast and tell the patient she has a benign tumor—unknown to the doctor the patient has a fatal malignant tumor elsewhere in the body. Unfortunately both doctor and patient develop false security . . .

"Often while making a biopsy the malignant tumor is cut across which tends to spread or accelerate the growth. Needle biopsies can accomplish the same tragic results."[129]

Fred Rohe reported the following on biopsies:

"In 1978 the Germans completed a seven-year study of biopsies and needle biopsies on women with breast cancer. They found that biopsies shortened the lives of the women considerably as compared with the control group that did not have biopsies (malignancies established by pathology reports)."[129]

Dr. Alan Cantwell added:

"Although doctors realize a healthy immune system is the body's best defense against cancer and AIDS, it is ironic to realize that the treatment of cancer is often chemotherapy, which is injurious to the immune system . . . statistics are not compiled of cancer patients dying as a direct result of cancer chemotherapy, and radiation."[102]

And Dr. Dick Richards has admitted:

"It is no longer a rarity to find patients at autopsy who have died not of their cancers, but of the means used for treating them. This is not a theory. It is already a matter of widespread medical record. Opinion could quite reasonably see this state of affairs as legalized manslaughter. It is unthinkable that such an untenable situation would have been reached. Yet it exists."[13]

This book cannot, by itself, start a long overdue change in cancer treatment regulations and provisions for alternative therapies. It can awaken and inform only one person at a time. Thus it is to you, my reader, that I give the responsibility of carrying the information provided here to your neighbors, political representatives, newspapers and physicians, in order that some of the suggested changes can start to take root. Who must do the hard tasks? Whoever can!

If one *protected* alternative cancer clinic in the United States or Canada results from this book—because one physician, one attorney, one political leader, one media advocate, makes it happen—then this book will have accomplished its goal. From that model clinic can come thousands of clinics and healing therapies. Only one is needed.

For poorer cities, it is a golden opportunity for revitalization that is being offered here. It would require great civic support and citizen courage, but to establish a viable alternative cancer therapy protected by law, where desperate patients could be healed of cancer, would be historic and would inundate an impoverished town, city or state with visitors bringing money and energy.

The great problem is mass communication. A media afraid to tackle so fundamental an issue as a corrupt health system means that the democratic values of the nation are in jeopardy. Media critic Ben Bagdikian reminds us:

"The root process of peaceful and appropriate change begins with the right of the aggrieved to be heard, thus presenting the best evidence of the need for change. . . . The media are crucial to this process. If the media do not report malfunctions of the system, the unheard cries never become a social fact. Or if the public, sensing the need for change, has opinions that go unreported, no mechanism exists for consensus to evolve . . . the result is apathy or violence, both of which are subversive of democracy."[130]

When it comes to reporting news on cancer, the media is essentially as controlled as any totalitarian state. This statement is hard to believe, but a number of journalists know it to be true.

On December 1, 1977, NBC aired a news report on the work of those who had developed the cancer serum (Glover, Deaken, Livingston-Wheeler, etc.). According to Dr. Robert E. Netterberg and Robert Taylor's *The Cancer Conspiracy:*

"NBC provided scientific facts that the possibility for a universal cancer vaccine exists. Tests on animals were 70% effective."[56]

NCI ignored the nationwide report, based on months of careful checking by the network. UPI and AP, the press syndicates, refused to send out a story based on NBC's report. Dr. Netterberg contacted AP (Associated Press) to find out why. He was told that "all cancer stories had to be cleared from the science editing department of the AP in New York."

All cancer stories had to be cleared by one group in New York City where the American Cancer Society and Memorial Sloan-Kettering had virtual control of all policies relating to cancer. All cancer stories for all the citizens of America had to be "approved" just as all treatments had to be "approved" and by the same people?!

Whatever happened to Freedom of the Press? Whatever happened to the Constitution of the United States of America? Who empowered Mary Lasker and her friends as official press

153

censor for anything relating to cancer? Nobody. And that power can be taken from them. If our journalists ever get up off their knees.

The great editor of *The New Yorker* magazine, William Shawn, once wrote, "To be silent when something is going on that shouldn't be going on would be cowardly."[130]

Something *The New Yorker* and the rest of the New York media should have spotted and condemned occurred in 1980. One of their own, *Newsweek* columnist Jane Bryant Quinn, was used to do a hatchet job on a rival of the American Cancer Society. Here are the dirty details, exemplifying how the cancer establishment uses a variety of weapons to keep its "gross public deception" and its criminal medical procedures from being openly examined or changed.

Remember Albert Szent-Gyorgyi, the 1937 Nobel Prize Winner for discovering Vitamin C and the "father of electrobiology" for his famous 1941 speech (chapter six)? He was still doing research in the 1970s, but because most biologists were stuck at the molecular level and Szent-Gyorgyi was "amid the dance of electrons . . . a dimension below the molecules" (Ralph Moss, *Free Radical,* 1988), Szent-Gyorgyi couldn't get any funding. The National Cancer Institute had rejected his grant requests four times (a Nobel Prize winner being refused by the cancer bureaucrats!). So Szent-Gyorgyi hooked up with a private foundation which began soliciting funds for his research.

The National Foundation for Cancer Research (NFCR) was established in 1974 and by 1979-80 was pulling in several million dollars a year. This obviously irritated the American Cancer Society (ACS) which saw a powerful rival emerging. One ACS official, Congdon Woods, complained, "They are competing with us in fund-raising and they're creating a great deal of confusion" (*Science* magazine, February 9, 1979).

On December 22, 1980, during the NFCR's fund-raising campaign, Jane Bryant Quinn's column in *Newsweek* was used to attack NFCR's credibility. Titled "Look Before Giving," it was a devastating blow to the reputation of the new cancer organization. Quinn whined that the NFCR had "no connection to the American Cancer Society or to any government agency." So what? Had American cancer research reached the point where only the ACS and NCI could do cancer research? Quinn also mentioned that NFCR wasn't approved by the non-profit standards organizations. Neither was the American Cancer Society, but Quinn conveniently forgot to mention that. She also omitted that a Nobel Prize winner of Szent-Gyorgyi's stature was the primary recipient of NFCR's funds or that other respected scientists received grants.

NFCR sued *Newsweek* but the national weekly magazine threw its army of lawyers at NFCR. Five years of legal frustration finally brought NFCR a short item in *Newsweek* (December 2, 1985) and no admission of error by the publishers.

The New York media could have investigated what was behind the charges. *Newsweek* or its owner, *The Washington Post* (famous for exposing the Watergate coverup), could have "looked into" the history of the ACS and its links with the other elements of the cancer establishment—drug companies, FDA, AMA, NCI, etc. They chose not to investigate.

NFCR in time grew conservative, moving away from financing revolutionary "bio-electronic" cancer research and more toward traditional cancer researchers. Many such scientists received grants not only from NFCR but also ACS and NCI. The cancer revolution that "almost was" petered out. Szent-Gyorgyi died in 1986. Yet, for a short time, the ACS was obviously worried. Large funds had been made available for non-traditional research. *Newsweek* and Jane Bryant Quinn (now an occasional TV commentator as well as a newspaper and magazine columnist) had struck the blow which knocked the anti-establishment cancer foundation off-course. Millions of lives might have been saved if this event had not happened—if the non-traditional approach had grown, evolved into investigating the suppressed cancer cures, and contributed to the development of the new clinical treatments which ACS, FDA and others were keeping from the American and Canadian public.

Dr. Robert C. Atkins defined the issue confronting the people of North America most bluntly in his 1988 book, *Dr Atkins' Health Revolution* (Houghton Mifflin, Boston, 1988). It is unfortunate that *Newsweek, The Washington Post* and

155

other leading media cannot find the courage to inform their readers of what now threatens their health and their constitutional rights. Dr. Atkins:

> "There have already been *many* cancer cures, and all have been ruthlessly and systematically suppressed with a Gestapo-like thoroughness by the cancer establishment. The cancer establishment is the not-too-shadowy association of the American Cancer Society, the leading cancer hospitals, the National Cancer Institute, and the FDA. The shadow part is the fact that these respected institutions are very much dominated by members and friends of members of the pharmaceutical industry, which profits so incredibly much from our profession-wide obsession with chemotherapy . . .

> "The health field is the only field where inequity, conflict of interest, and gross public deception can remain unchecked. After all, the people in the FDA and in all the branches of government that deal with health come from the same orthodox school of thought as the heads of the AMA . . .

> "The damage done to the body by an unsuccessful course of chemotherapy is often so great that the patient's immune system never recovers sufficiently for him to stand a fighting chance . . .

> "Chemotherapy, when it has no chance, or only a remote chance, to work is at best stupid and at worst criminal."[94]

On behalf of 10,000 Americans and countless others worldwide who die of cancer this week, packed into the cancer wards where surgery, chemotherapy and radiation comprise a 20th century conveyer belt to torture, disfigurement and death, I implore you, the reader, to become part of the solution by supporting nonconventional cancer centers and patient choice.

Even the U.S. Congress' biased OTA (Office of Technology Assessment) 1990 report on unconventional cancer treatments acknowledged that Congress ought to "determine whether there are not better laws and regulations that would enhance both consumer protection and freedom of choice in the interests of Americans with cancer."

Chapter Twelve

# Something Wrong/Something to be Fixed

*"There is one thing I do not underestimate, and that is the—to me—amazing and unexpected intuition of the American public."*

The great Swiss psychologist,
Carl Jung

*"Common talk in the checkout line . . . ultimately translates into politics. A good politician is one who can voice aloud and clearly what people know to be their own private resentments. Politicians win when they convert such discontent into issues."*

The great political journalist
Theodore H. White

America is where the change must come. It is where the medical monopoly has operated most criminally. It is where the murder and the attempted murder of those who oppose the existing drug medicine has produced a climate of fear reminiscent of the worst totalitarian terror tactics. It is where Benjamin Rush's warning of an "undercover dictatorship" has come to be. It is where censorship and book burning has blatantly occurred and few speak out, even though the most precious of the nation's Constitutional Rights—freedom of speech—has been threatened. It is where Congress has been intimidated. Robert G. Houston has warned us (*Cancer Scandal* video):

"Probably today, more than any time in modern history there is a strike force, a hit force, that is coordinated by some of the agencies—the FDA, the National Cancer Institute, the Post Office, the Justice Department—and now the Narc squads too. The Drug Enforcement Agency is involved in it, working hand in hand with the FDA to raid doctor's offices, to raid health food stores, to harass, intimidate and to show the power of the gun. . . . This is such a profound violation of rights . . . so characteristic of totalitarian terror tactics. There is evidence that this is all coordinated in a massive movement to stamp out all alternative doctors. . . . At least 50 and probably more like a 100 doctors in the past two years have undergone such treatment."[26]

Dr. Robert C. Atkins provides additional testimony against this enemy that has brought the Gestapo to birth within America:

"There's a war going on. . . . The War Against Quackery is a carefully orchestrated, heavily endowed campaign sponsored by extremists holding positions of power in the orthodox hierarchy . . .

The multimillion-dollar campaign against quackery was never meant to root out incompetent doctors; *it was, and is, designed specifically to destroy alternative medicine.* . . . The millions were raised and spent because orthodox medicine sees alternative, *drugless* medicine as a real threat to its economic power.

"And right they are. . . . The majority of the drug houses will not survive."[94]

Many people sense what is happening. They know the medical profession is totally outside any decision-making process of the average citizen. They may not talk about it openly. But the public perceives that there is a public health crisis and that money is only one factor. Congress knows as well. Knows deep down in its gut and yet treads carefully, afraid to step on the powerful toes. Lots of us know. And the murmurings will grow.

"Patients go into a hospital scared to death, as well they might. These people in white coats are not necessarily looking out for his interests."

Patrick McGrady, Jr.
*Cancer Scandal* video[26]

"One of the side effects of X-ray . . . and chemotherapy is the suppression . . . of the patient's immunological

158

defenses. . . . A simple cold often leads to death from pneumonia."

G. Edward Griffin, "The Hoax of<br>the Proven Cancer Cure"[131]

"The hearings have revealed police-state tactics . . . possibly perjured testimony to gain a conviction . . . intimidation and gross disregard for Constitutional Rights. . . . The FDA is bent on using snooping gear to pry and invade."

U.S. Senator Edward Long<br>Hearings, U.S. Senate[17]

"Maybe the raising of millions of dollars of funds for charitable projects has become a 'racket'. . . . Maybe we should investigate the American Cancer Society's operations."

U.S. Representative Roland Libonati[7]

"If we are just going to be brokering out these grants on the basis of who has published a paper that passes some peer group as the only criteria, then I dare say we will be fumbling in this morass of inconclusive research forever and ever."

U.S. Senator John Melcher[7]

"On two occasions Gerson became violently ill. . . . Lab tests showed . . . arsenic in his urine. Some of Gerson's best case histories mysteriously disappeared from his files . . . Gerson was invited on a talk show by host Long John Nebel. . . . Nebel was fired the very next day and the radio network was threatened by the AMA."

Norman Fritz[35]

"One death from poisoning, and one from being run down by an automobile, both victims being physicians of distinction and prominent in the advocacy of the Koch treatment. Mail has been opened . . . Dr. Koch himself was the target of at least 13 unsuccessful attempts on his life."

M. Layne[31]

"Dr. Ivy . . . sent his article (on Krebiozen) to one medical journal after another. . . . The journals accepted his article for publication, only to return it with apologies . . . Dr. Ivy was informed that the publishers were told by the AMA headquarters they would lose all their revenue from pharmaceutical advertising if they published Ivy's article . . .

"I went to the Main Branch of the New York Public Library,

159

the largest in the world. The librarian-in-charge advised me that . . . the author 'went against' the AMA and it was decided that this book (K-Krebiozen) was to be 'taboo'."

Herbert Bailey[132]

"Bruce Halstead, M.D. . . . was given a five-year jail sentence . . . . The crime? Dr. Halstead prescribed and sold to several of his cancer patients some herbal remedies . . . a rather onerous California law . . . forbids a doctor to treat a cancer patient with anything other than chemotherapy, radiation or surgery."

Dr. Robert C. Atkins[94]

This is a criminal conspiracy. To whitewash it with any other name is to lie in the face of evil. Any of the actions cited above, if not initiated or sanctioned by powerful groups with substantial influence in government, would be quickly met with law enforcement and media counteraction. The absence of such a response signifies the approval or acquiescence of those elected to defend the Constitution. The seriousness of the situation cannot be overemphasized.

Fundamental change will not be easy. It will require substantial citizen participation. It will require a media that educates and investigates. It will require political leadership.

The stakes are nothing less than the survival of the nation because continuation of the status quo—ignoring the fact of an "undercover dictatorship"—threatens not only the health of the nation but also the political principles and Constitutional protections upon which America is based. Again, the issue is democracy and citizen rights—choice—as opposed to tyranny, subversion, censorship and the murder of millions.

"Five hours after presenting a lecture on cancer before an audience of about 400 in Los Angeles, the windshield was shot out of my car on the road back to San Francisco. The next night the glass window in the tailgate was shot out."

Ernest J. Krebs[133]

"One doctor . . . J. W. Kannel, saved a young girl. . . . She had hopeless cancer of the spleen. . . . One shot of Glyoxylide, and she became well (in 1943, and still alive in 1983). . . . Kannel was barred from all hospitals in Fort

Wayne. . . . The FDA had Koch arrested and thrown into an incredibly filthy jail in Florida in 1942."

Wayne Martin,
*We Can Do Without Heart Attacks, 1983*[31]

"It was in 1936 that I copyrighted *Cancer, Its Cause and Control*. They forced me to serve a whole year in jail. . . . When I had everything ready to put out a third edition, they notified me in no uncertain terms 'Unless you stop . . . . We will snatch you . . . and do a lobotomy on you.'"

Emerson Hartman,
*Cancer News Journal*, 1977[134]

"Dr. Wilhelm Hueper, retired chief of NCI's environmental cancer section, prophesied in the early 1960s that 'Chemical technology is biological dynamite.'. . . In a 1966 book, according to a review published July 19, 1967 in the *British Medical Journal,* Dr. Hueper 'assembled an impressive body of evidence which shows that the occupational and environmental causes are of equal if not more importance' than cigarettes in the genesis of lung cancer."

Peter Barry Chowka.
"The Cancer Charity Ripoff"[37]

"When I submitted that manuscript for clearance, I was called . . . in to the office of my (NCI) director. He said, 'Now, the high medical official of the Atomic Energy Commission objects against that. . . . You shall omit that. . . . My studies on occupational cancer in industries was forcefully and abruptly brought to a halt . . . by an order of the Surgeon General. (This followed) a protest to the Public Health Service by (an) industry alleging that my activities were detrimental to their interests. . . . I was forbidden (by the Public Health Service) to contact, thereafter, state health departments and industrial concerns on all matters of occupational cancer. (I was) to discontinue all field work."

Dr. Wilhelm C. Hueper, Chief,
Environmental Cancer Section NCI[135]

"Dr. Emanuel Revici developed an entirely new approach to the treatment of disease, and proceeded to use it to cure cancer. He is still doing it at age 92. He published an 800 page book in 1961. Of 10,000 copies, the government burned 7,000, saying they were 'dangerous.' It is a superb book in which, 30 years before a Nobel Prize went to someone else, he discovered Leukotrienes. Also the oncogene. Also Prostaglandins. Also Pleomorphic Bacteria. Wouldn't it have been wonderful if he and Rife could have worked together? Also a complete Lipidic system in the body. A concept of a "hierarchy of levels." A concept of dualism—anabolic versus catabolic. He also knew of free oxygen radicals. He is still (at 92) restoring terminal cancer patients and AIDS patients to normalcy."

1989 communication from one of
Dr. Revici's patients

"We were told that owners of drugstores, a vital outlet for paperbacks, had been notified that any druggist who displayed my book on his paperback racks, would not receive any more prescriptions from members of the AMA."

Glenn Kittler[136]

"There is not one, but many cures for cancer available. But they are all being systematically suppressed by the ACS, the NCI and the major oncology centers. They have too much of a vested interest in the status quo."

Robert C. Atkins, M.D.[7]

"The people think the FDA is protecting them. It isn't. What the FDA is doing and what the public *thinks* it's doing are as different as night and day . . ."

FDA Commissioner Herbert Ley[17]

"I never have and never will approve a 'new drug' to an individual, but only to a large pharmaceutical firm with unlimited finances.

Dr. J. Richard Crout,
Director of Bureau of Drugs, FDA,
quoted in 1982[137]

Only if alternative cancer centers, protected by law, are established which use a wide variety of now illegal *but effective* cancer therapies will this terrible crime end. When such cancer centers become reality, cancer will become an illness which can be easily treated and cured. But until the American people stand up for their freedom and do something more than give lip service to alternative cancer centers, we all must share the judgment of history because we are permitting this monstrous crime perpetrated by vested interests, profiteers and a brainwashed medical elite.

"A recent Associated Press poll found that over half of the American public want alternative cancer clinics in the USA whether the medical establishment approves or not. Most of the unfair attacks on alternative cancer treatments . . . are carried out by Medical Associations rather than Federal or State Government Agencies, but they would be ineffective if they were not supported by government funds and influence."

Professor Harold S. Ladas
Hunter College, City University
of New York[138]

"Many cancer victims have testified that they have received benefit and, in some cases, have been cured by a variety of treatments . . . Why were they not studied, objectively, by established cancer research organizations? . . . Do they really want to cure cancer? Everybody but the patient is doing well in the cancer business . . . What little cancer auditing that has been done was mostly by those who were in some manner connected with the cancer business. Does a company treasurer audit his own books?"

Richard Ericson, *Cancer Treatment:
Why So Many Failures?*[139]

"And what of the powerful effect of . . . EDTA in the prevention of cancer? Walter Blummer, in his remarkable paper, showed that patients given 10 to 15 treatments of EDTA—but no other recommendations about cessation of smoking, exercise, diet, vitamin/mineral supplementation etc.—showed a remarkable resistance to the development of cancer when checked 18 years later. (*Ninety Percent Reduction in Cancer Mortality After Chelation Therapy with EDTA,* Blummer, W., MD and Cranton, E., MD, *J. Advancement Med,* Vol 2, 1989.)"

"Why don't medical schools teach this? Has it anything to do with the desires of the drug companies, which finance the majority of basic and advanced drug research in these institutions?"

E. W. McDonagh, DO[140]

"According to medical historian Brandon Reines, proponents of animal research have re-written medical history for political reasons . . . Dr. Reines has found that most major advances in areas such as heart disease and cancer have developed from human clinical investigation . . . Are we wasting billions of dollars on inappropriate animal research?"

A necessary tactic for the survival of animal research—a measure that, incidently, is decidedly anti-science—has been the silencing of its critics . . . Many research scientists . . . have been intimidated from speaking out."

*Medical Research Modernization*
*Committee Report,* May 1990[141]

"The IACVF (International Association of Cancer Victors and Friends) . . . tells of a raid against one of their public meetings by the Nassau County (NY) District Attorney, during which several people were arrested, handcuffed, and dragged away . . . Their homes were searched."

*Cancer Victors Journal*
March 1975[142]

Lorenzo Haché M.D. is a cancer surgeon in Quebec, Canada where the same type of oppressive political system dominates medicine as in the U.S.A. During court testimony against a nonconventional cancer treatment in 1989, Dr. Haché made the following incredible admission regarding his hospital's policy when dealing with a reluctant cancer patient who decided to cancel orthodox treatment in order to seek alternative therapy:

"We often send out police to locate such reluctant patients."

Christopher Bird, *The Life*
*and Trials of Gaston Naessens*[143]

"The Nuremberg Code, adopted after World War II, held that the patient 'should be so situated as to be able to exercise free power of choice, without the intervention of any element of force, fraud, deceit, duress, over-reaching or other ulterior form of constraint or coercion.'"

Ralph Moss, *The Cancer Industry*[144]

The right of the individual to elect freely the manner of his care in illness must be preserved."

Dwight D. Eisenhower, President,
United States of America, 1953-1961[145]

## Chapter Thirteen
# Avenging Angels

"There will be a medical edition of the Nuremberg Trials. The atrocities now being committed in the name of orthodox medicine, the suppression of life-giving scientific data, the needless loss of lives, mutilation of bodies, and excessive suffering . . . will not be tolerated. . . . Ultimately, these criminals and their political lackeys will be brought to trial . . ."

Dr. Bruce Halstead[146]

"Dr. Shirley and I go over the chemotherapy procedure for the last time. I will lose all my hair and menstrual periods may stop. . . . My cancer textbook tells me how important it is for the patient to receive the maximum dose of chemotherapy drugs each time. . . . I throw up every fifteen minutes. . . . Five hours. . . . Eight. . . . At eleven hours the sky is beginning to lighten, and I think the ordeal will have to end pretty soon. . . . After eighteen hours I stop vomiting. . . . I don't think I can go through this four more times. . . . Three days later, I am able to get up, shaky and depressed . . .

"The cancer returned. . . . They irradiated me, but in April, it was back again. . . . Sure, you'll lose your hair like you did before with chemotherapy, but it is only ten radiation treatments to the head. It couldn't be simpler. No one at the outpatient clinic tells me that radiation burns. My tongue, nose, throat and lungs feel like they have been scraped and salted . . .

"Now I am beginning chemotherapy . . . it isn't fair for a patient to have to watch such terrible things happen to her body without understanding they are going to happen. Methotrexate, one of the three chemotherapy drugs to be used, can damage the brain. But what a time to tell me—minutes before I am to receive the drug."

Dorothea Lynch (she died following<br>treatment while still in her thirties)[147]

"It took me shamefully long to realize that the methods we were all using were worthless failures . . .

"Looking around at the incessant horror of cancer, seeing people I know and care about suffer, not only from the disease but from the appalling methods being unsuccessfully used to treat them, one thing has become abundantly clear to me. There just is not time to wait for other ideas to die out. People in vast numbers are going through unutterable horrors to their deaths. The old ideas must get out of the way. There is no point in beating about the bush. Those who hold the other opinions are wrong. They and their ideas must go . . .

"The new and better ways *are* all available *now*. No one can do worse from them, and most do better. . . . It is no longer premature to claim that cancer really is a beaten disease."

Dr. Dick Richards<br>*The Topic of Cancer: When*<br>*the Killing Has to Stop*[13]

"Over 30 years ago urine tests began to be developed which could easily and effectively determine the presence of malignant tumors. . . . They measure the improvement or failure of improvement as treatment progresses. They can tell when and if a treatment being used is effective . . .

"Halting or stopping the malignant growth is relatively simple. The clinical problem in treating a cancer victim is clearing the body of accumulated toxins. The growth is usually stopped from within 3 hours to 12 days. . . . Then comes the long, laborious period of detoxication. This takes from 3 months to 12 months."

Dr. William D. Kelley<br>*One Answer to Cancer*[129]

# Appendix A
# An Open Letter to the Community on the Subject of Cancer

(This first appeared in the November 1, 1988 *Carmel Valley Sun;* written by Ralph Auer; reproduced with the permission of Ralph Auer.)

On January 31 of this year, the day after her fifty-sixth birthday, my wife lost her very courageous nine-year battle with breast cancer. Until a year and a half before her passing, we both believed early detection was important and, if caught early, breast cancer was nearly 100% curable through surgery, radiation therapy, chemotherapy, or a combination of the three. Not only were we deceived but, ironically, she will be counted as cured because she survived at least five years.

This year, the American Cancer Society will take in three hundred million dollars in charitable contributions. Last year the National Cancer Institute spent $1.4 billion of U.S. taxpayers' money; by 1993, that figure will go to $3.1 billion. We Americans are now spending between fifty and one hundred billion dollars each year on cancer research and therapy. To date, almost one trillion dollars has been spent on cancer research and treatment since the war on cancer was declared in 1971. Cancer has become a very big business in the United States, and someone has said that there are now more people making a living off cancer than there are people dying of cancer. I would add that some of these people are making a *very good* living.

On March 5, 1987, the American Cancer Society released the following statement to the Associated Press: "Caught early enough, breast cancer has cure rates approaching 100 percent." Less than a month ago, the retiring director of the National Cancer Institute, Vincent DeVita, stated in an interview on the MacNeil/Lehrer Newshour that when he came to

NCI eight years ago, one in three cancer patients were being cured; now, one in two cancer patients are being cured. The American Cancer Society has been advertising continually in the media to tell all women over thirty-five to get a mammogram because "early" breast cancer is so curable. Unfortunately, the information is not true. During the past several years, a large number of physicians and scientists have been making statements about the lack of progress of the war on cancer and the lack of effectiveness of the approved therapies in curing cancer—statements which the cancer establishment chooses to ignore. Here are only a few such comments;

1. "Progress in the war on cancer has been limited and overstated." (General Accounting Office report to Congress, 1987.)

2. "These data, taken alone, provide no evidence that some 35 years of intense and growing efforts to improve the treatment of cancer have had much overall effect on the most fundamental measure of clinical outcome—death. Indeed, with respect to cancer as a whole, we have slowly lost ground, as shown by the rise in age-adjusted mortality rates in the entire population." (Bailar and Smith in the May 8, 1986 issue of the *New England Journal of Medicine*.)

3. "The cancer cure rate for the overall population has remained virtually unchanged since 1930." (Congressional hearings, 1977.)

4. "Despite improved surgical techniques, advanced methods in radiotherapies, and widespread use of chemotherapies, breast cancer mortality has not changed in the past 70 years." (Thomas I. Dao, M.D., Department of Breast Surgery, Roswell Park Memorial Institute, on the occasion of the Institute's 75th Anniversary in 1975.)

5. "The evidence that breast cancer is incurable is overwhelming. The philosophy of breast cancer screening is based on wishful thinking that early cancer is curable cancer, though no one knows what is 'early'. . . . Survival rates are little affected by any of the current methods used, whether it be radical or simple mastectomy, with or without radiation, and with or without chemotherapy." (Dr. Petr Skrabanek, *Lancet 2316,* 1985.)

6. "Mammography is very expensive; $195,000 per cancer detected . . ." (Dr. Petr Skrabanek, *Lancet 2316,* 1985.)

7. ". . . five-year survival rates don't represent anything close to a cure." (John A. McDougall, M.D., *McDougall's Medicine: A Challenging Second Opinion,* New Century Publishers, 1985.)

8. "The Cancer Society fails to tell us that the 'improved' survival rates seen over the past eighty years for most cancers is largely the result of early detection, not more effective treatment. Finding the cancer earlier does allow more people to live five years from the time of diagnosis. Thus, more people will fit the definition of 'cured.' However, in most cases early detection does not change the day of death, but only the length of time a person is aware that he or she has cancer. Under the circumstances, the real beneficiaries of early detection are the providers of health care, who now have a longer time in which to treat the victims before they die. This means they can charge for more doctor's visits, more procedures, more tests, and longer hospital stays. The American Cancer Society proclaims great success in the treatment of cancer. The best that can be said for this claim is that the Society has put hope up for sale. Unfortunately, to date, it has been selling mostly false hope." (John A McDougall, M.D., *McDougall's Medicine: A Challenging Second Opinion,* New Century Publishers, 1985.)

Fortunately, there are alternatives.

Ralph Auer

---

In 1989 Ralph Auer moved from California back to Boulder, Colorado where he had lived for thirteen years with his wife while she was alive. In September of 1989, he spent $1500 for a full page ad in the local newspaper, the *Daily Camera.* Soon a firestorm of denunciations appeared from several members of the Colorado cancer establishment. The next day the newspaper carried a story with the headline, "Cancer ad raises a ruckus." But many citizens applauded, calling Ralph Auer or approaching him on the street or at public meetings after a subsequent story and interview included his picture. His new neighbors thanked him for his public service. One reader wrote to the newspaper and reminded them, "Our democracy was founded on dissent."

Ralph Auer is still available to talk and provide information. He still cares and he is still raising a ruckus. His new address is:

Ralph Auer
840 11th St.
Boulder, CO 80302

# Appendix B
# Selections from the Fitzgerald Report

The following appeared in the *Congressional Record Appendix* on August 3, 1953. It is the report of Ben Fitzgerald, special counsel to the Senate Committee on Interstate and Foreign Commerce. He concludes that there is a conspiracy by the cancer establishment.

"A Report to the Senate Interstate Commerce Committee on the Need for Investigation of Cancer Research Organizations . . .

"There is reason to believe that the AMA has been hasty, capricious, arbitrary, and outright dishonest . . .

"Being vitally interested and having tried to listen and observe closely, it is my profound conviction that this substance krebiozen is one of the most promising materials yet isolated for the management of cancer. It is biologically active. I have gone over the records of 530 cases, most of them conducted at a distance from Chicago, by unbiased cancer experts and clinics. In reaching my conclusions I have of course discounted my own lay observations and relied mostly on the opinions of qualified cancer research workers and ordinary experienced physicians.

"I have concluded that in the value of present cancer research, this substance and the theory behind it deserves the most full and complete and scientific study. Its value in the management of the cancer patient has been demonstrated in a sufficient number and percentage of cases to demand further work.

"Behind and over all this is the weirdest conglomeration of corrupt motives, intrigue, selfishness, jealousy, obstruction, and conspiracy that I have ever seen.

"Dr. Andrew C. Ivy, who has been conducting research upon this drug, is absolutely honest intellectually, scientifically, and in every other way. Moreover, he appears to be one of the most competent and unbiased cancer experts that I have ever come in contact with, having served on the board of the American Cancer Society and the American Medical Association, and in that capacity having been called upon to evaluate various types of cancer therapy. Dr. George O. Stoddard, president of the University of Illinois, in assisting in the cessation of Dr. Ivy's research on cancer at the University of Illinois, and in recommending the abolishment of the latter's post as vice-president of that institution, has, in my opinion, shown attributes of intolerance for scientific research in general . . .

"Now, passing on to another institution, I have very carefully studied the court records of three cases tried in the Federal and State courts of Dallas, Tex. A running fight has been going on between officials, especially Dr. Morris Fishbein, of the American Medical Association through the journal of that organization, and the Hoxsey Cancer Clinic. Dr. Fishbein contended that the medicines employed by the Hoxsey Cancer Clinic had no therapeutic value: that it was run by a quack and a charlatan . . .

"It is interesting to note that in the trial court, before Judge Atwell, who had an opportunity to hear the witnesses in two different trials, it was held that the so-called Hoxsey method of treating cancer was in some respects superior to that of X-ray, radium, and surgery and did have therapeutic value . . .

"The defense admitted that Hoxsey could cure external cancer but contended that his medicines for internal cancer had no therapeutic value. The jury, after listening to leading pathologists, radiologists, physicians, surgeons, and scores of witnesses, a great number of whom had never been treated by any physician or surgeon except the treatment received at the Hoxsey Cancer Clinic, concluded that Dr. Fishbein was wrong: that his published statements were false, and that the Hoxsey method of treating cancer did have therapeutic value.

"In this litigation the Government of the United States, as

172

well as Dr. Fishbein, brought to the court the leading medical scientists, including pathologists and others skilled in the treatment of cancer. They came from all parts of the country. It is significant to note that a great number of these doctors admitted that X-ray therapy could cause cancer . . .

"Report of Dr. Miley of a survey made by Dr. Stanley Reimann (in charge of tumor research and pathology, Gotham Hospital). . . . Dr. Reimann's report on cancer cases in Pennsylvania over a long period of time showed that those who received no treatment lived a longer period than those that received surgery, radium, or X-ray. . . . The survey also showed that following the use of radium and X-ray much more harm than good was done to the average cancer patient . . .

"There is a report from another source in which Dr. Feinblatt, for 6 years pathologist of the Memorial (Sloan-Kettering) Hospital, New York, reported that the Memorial Hospital had originally given X-ray and radium treatment before and after radical operations for breast malignancy. These patients did not long survive, so X-ray and radium were given after surgery only. These patients lived a brief time only, after omitting all radiation, patients lived the longest of all . . .

"Dr. Herman Joseph Muller, Nobel Prize winner, a world-renowned scientist, has stated the medical profession is permanently damaging the American life stream through the unwise use of X-rays. There is no dosage of X-ray so low as to be without risk of producing harmful mutations.

"The attention of the committee is invited to the request made by Senator Elmer Thomas following an investigation made by the Senator of the Hoxsey Cancer Clinic under date of February 25, 1947, and addressed to the Surgeon General, Public Health Department, Washington, D.C., wherein he sought to enlist the support of the Federal Government to make an investigation and report. No such investigation was made. In fact, every effort was made to avoid and evade the investigation by the Surgeon General's office. The record will reveal that this clinic did furnish 62 complete case histories, including pathology, names of hospitals, physicians, etc. in 1945. Again, in June 1950, 77 case histories, which included the names of the patients, pathological reports in many instances, and in the absence thereof, the names of the pathologists, hospitals, and physicians who had treated these patients before being treated at the Hoxsey Cancer Clinic. The Council of National Cancer Institute, without investigation, in October 1950, refused to order an investigation. The record in the Federal court discloses that this agency of the Federal Government took sides and sought in every way to hinder, suppress, and restrict this institution in their treatment of cancer . . .

"Among the numerous foundations and clinics which profess to possess a remedy for the treatment of cancer is the Lincoln Foundation of Medford, Mass., which has been the particular target of the AMA . . .

"I have approached this problem with an open mind. Recognizing the importance of men skilled in the science of medicine, who are best informed, if not qualified, on the question of cancer, its causes and treatment, I directed my attention to the propaganda by the American Medical Association and the American Cancer Society to the effect, namely, 'that radium, X-ray therapy, and surgery are the only recognized treatments for cancer.'

"Is there any dispute among recognized medical scientists in America and elsewhere in the world on the use of radium and X-ray therapy in the treatment of cancer? The answer is definitely 'Yes.' There is a division of opinion on the use of radium and X-ray. Both agencies are destructive, not constructive. In the alleged destruction of the abnormal, outlaw, or cancer cells both X-ray therapy and radium destroy normal tissue and normal cells. Recognized medical authorities in America and elsewhere state positively that X-ray therapy can cause cancer in and of itself. Documented cases are available . . .

"If radium, X-ray, or surgery or either of them is the complete answer, then the greatest hoax of the age is being perpetrated upon the people by the continued appeal for funds for further research. If neither X-ray, radium, or surgery is the complete answer to this dreaded disease, and I submit that it is not, then what is the plain duty of society? Should we stand still? Should we sit idly by and count the number of physicians, surgeons, and cancerologists who are not only divided but who, because of fear or favor, are forced to line up with the so-called accepted view of the American Medical Association, or should this committee make a full-scale investigation of the organized effort to hinder, suppress, and restrict the free flow of drugs which allegedly have proven successful in cases where clinical records, case history, pathological reports, and X-ray photographic proof, together with the alleged cured patients, are available?

"Accordingly, we should determine whether existing agencies, both public and private, are engaged and have pursued a policy of harrassment, ridicule, slander, and libelous attacks on others sincerely engaged in stamping out this curse of mankind. Have medical associations, through their officers, agents, servants and employees engaged in this practice? My investigation to date should convince this committee that a conspiracy does exist to stop the free flow and use of drugs in interstate commerce which allegedly have solid therapeutic value. Public and private funds have been thrown around like confetti at a country fair to close up and destroy clinics, hospitals, and scientific research laboratories which do not conform to the viewpoint of medical associations.

"How long will the American people take this? . . .

"What is the duty of this committee and the members thereof? Your first duty, of course, is to do right. Properly considered, that is your only duty. In doing right, however, you owe a duty to the American people. In upholding the law and enacting legislation for the people of America, we look first to the instrument of our creation as a representative form of government. Those powers not specifically conferred upon the Federal Government and denied to the States are reserved either to the States or to the people. Thus, the founding fathers very wisely created an area of freedom in which free men shall function.

"It is in this area set aside by the fathers of our Republic that people have the right to own property, transact business, build up a system of free enterprise without hindrance, harrassment, or abuse of either the Government, State or Federal, or of other citizens, however powerful, so long as the people so engaged do not trespass upon the rights of others. This is the basic concept of liberty functioning in America. It may be said to be a reservoir of freedom. In this area we have mingled our money and blood with the races of mankind. We have demonstrated our ability to live together peacefully and happily, although we represent most of the races, most of the colors and most of the creeds. This was an innovation and a new experiment to the peoples of the Old World.

"Out of and from this area has sprung the noblest dream and saintliest purposes of mankind—purposes so strong and vital that it has become the envy and admiration of a waiting world. People look longingly to the shores of America and desire to make this their asylum of escape and hope for the future. It is more than a dream. It is a reality. While we have not solved all the problems of mankind, we have at least provided a sanctuary and the instruments of government, if properly guarded against the abuse of selfish men and organizations who would bend it to suit their purposes, which could live for centuries to come . . .

"We are under a compelling moral obligation . . . to the untold millions of cancer sufferers throughout the world to carry on this investigation. We cannot do otherwise.

"Respectfully submitted.

"BENEDICT F. FITZGERALD, Jr.
    Special Counsel"

# Appendix C
# The Awful Truth

The American public, its representatives in Congress, the civil servants who administer the laws from the government agencies, and the Supreme Court which interprets the laws passed by Congress, have made assumptions about the practice of cancer medicine and cancer science which are untrue. As a result, all the nation's laws regarding the treatment of cancer and the protection of cancer patients are fundamentally flawed. Instead of insuring that the best cancer therapies are available for the American public, the lawmakers and the law enforcers have accomplished the opposite. They have limited the choice of cancer therapies to the worst and the most dangerous while protecting a small group of cancer scientists and cancer physicians (oncologists, radiologists and surgeons) who have a vested interest in preventing any deep uprooting of the existing structure. The result, hard as it may be for the American public to admit, is institutionalized murder for profit and/or prestige. The cause is simply human greed, career ambition, status-seeking, narrow-minded thinking, old-boy network elitism, political expediency and just plain stupidity. Plus the failure of Congress, the Media and the American people to be courageous and end the massacre of the innocent.

Irwin D. Bross, Ph.D., former Director of Biostatistics at Roswell Park Memorial Institute for Cancer Research blew away large chunks of the wall protecting the cancer experts and policy makers in the two publications cited at the end of Chapter Five.[148, 149]

Bross convincingly showed with disciplined scientific studies that the animal model system is essentially worthless and that it perpetuates scientific fraud, but is vigorously defended because it is "so highly profitable to universities and research institutions." Bross also revealed how results in ani-

177

mal trials were used to justify new human trials when previous human trials already had proved a drug worthless (which shows to what absurd lengths the political scientists will go for the sake of their ambitions and despite the cost in human lives). Bross thus exposed the corruption and evil which operated at the high "grantsmanship" levels of the cancer establishment.

Bross made a particular point of denouncing the drug 5-FU, which has been widely used for 30 years because there was a perception that the American Cancer Society owned a percentage of the patent. According to Bross, "this may explain why many grant requests included use of the drug." 5-FU is still being used today on cancers despite 30 years of experiments that have shown its ineffectiveness and its extreme toxicity.

Bross reports that two and a half *decades* ago the dirty little secrets about 5-FU were being covered up at NCI (just as they still are):

> "Chemotherapeutic agents such as 5-FU were far more effective against the patient's white blood cell system and other host defense systems than against the cancer, so the high doses were counter-productive. When our studies using surface models showed this, the NCI bureaucrat . . . was furious, and NCI did not renew our contract . . . "

Bross argued that studies clearly proved that NCI dogmas relating to chemotherapy were false and had no scientific basis, yet continue to the present day and cause "unnecessary suffering and even death for . . . human cancer patients."

Just as the Bross revelations ripped a gigantic hole in the cancer establishment's wall in 1988 and 1989, another explosion tore apart another section of the barrier, exposing to public view equally dirty secrets. Evelleen Richards, Senior Lecturer in the Department of Science and Technology Studies at the University of Woolongong, New South Wales, Australia, authored "The Politics of Therapeutic Evaluation" which in 1988 appeared in a London Sociology Journal.[150]

By 1990, the article was being cited in the AMA's monthly journal, being studied by Congressmen and their aides in Washington, D.C., being referenced in a London newspaper article questioning the corruption in the American cancer establishment, and being examined by American attornies preparing to attack the cozy cancer racket in the courts.

Professor Richards provided an exhaustive, scholarly dissection of how the American cancer elite rigged cancer trials in order to discredit and suppress nonconventional therapies which might threaten their positions and expertise. Professor Richards showed that the basis for the FDA's laws, supported by the Supreme Court's ruling, was fundamentally flawed because the *assumption of unbiased professionals* determining "safety and effectiveness" was simply untrue! Professor Richards convincingly established that the professionals were biased. Their tests were rigged. Hundreds of thousands of desperate cancer patients were dying annually in the United States alone because a small group of cancer scientists and cancer doctors were engaged in conspiratorial activities to keep a lucrative monopoly for themselves. The collusion even involved the prestigious New England Journal of Medicine which bent the scientific rules of fair play when it served the interests of the old-boy network of toxic drug experts.

Professor Richards called for "consumer choice and market forces" to be given a role in determining what therapies could be permitted. The professor's revelations made it clear that Congress, the Courts and the Media had been asleep on the job while a small band of self-interested bureaucrats and cancer specialists had committed horrible crimes against cancer patients worldwide.

Professor Richards stated:

"medical authority is . . . clearly political in nature . . . innovations are only acceptable to the extent that they do not threaten the existing power position of the profession."

"the very organization and structure of professionally endorsed cancer research and treatment functions to exclude unconventional treatments."

"this implies a radical review of the expert's role in therapeutic evaluation. It also opens the way to an active and acknowledged evaluative role for non-experts, for patients and the public at large in the processes of assessment and decision-making."

The revelations of Dr. Bross and Professor Richards make

it obvious that it is now time for a massive assault on the evil cancer empire of vested interests masquerading as public service. It is now time to expose the crimes, punish the ringleaders, and begin constructing an alternative system which permits physicians and other qualified healers a wider latitude in providing non-toxic and innovative therapies for cancer patients. If we fail to undertake this task, the very foundation of democracy could be threatened.

> "Inherent in the meaning of professionalism and the motives of its adherents is the negation of democracy itself, stemming from the incipient belief that the citizen, like the consumer, is incompetent to make important decisions affecting his life."
>
> Jethro Lieberman,
> *Tyranny of the Experts*

# Appendix D
# Go and Climb a Mountain

The story of German doctor Josef Issels demonstrates that the European cancer establishment has been just as corrupt as its American counterpart and just as opposed to alternative cancer therapies which work. Instead of putting the patient first and evaluating new approaches developed by doctors at the clinical level, the European cancer "authorities" chose to abuse their positions of power in order to remove those who questioned the standard approaches to cancer.

Dr. Josef Issels became convinced in the 1930s that it was an error to focus on just the tumor. Instead, Issels concentrated on the whole body. Using a variety of orthodox as well as alternative treatments, Issels got cures with terminal cancer patients which were *eight times* greater than the World Health Organization indicated was likely. These were with *verified* terminal cases of cancer.

Among the unusual methods employed by Dr. Issels was his insistence that infected teeth and tonsils had to be removed because they released poisons into the system which interfered with the body's resistance. Dr. Issels also used homeopathic remedies, a cancer vaccine developed by a renowned Austrian researcher, psychotherapy, neural therapy to reestablish the "electrical field" where old body scars had disturbed it, and treatments for "masked tuberculosis." Diet, fever therapy and oxygen-ozone therapy were also employed.

Dr. Issels recognized that cancer had to be researched in the treatment area, not just with mice in the laboratory. He wrote:

"Nor is it enough just to do research work with mice and other animals. Only by research on cancer patients in their sickbeds can we develop a new therapy. . . . Until now, the so-called 'incurable' patient has never been treated. He has been sent home to die with a few pain-killers. That is not treatment."

Issels opened a clinic for terminally ill cancer patients on September 14, 1951. The Ringberg Klinik in Rottach-Egern, Bavaria would become world famous, not only for Issels' success but because of the fury with which German, English and American cancer officials attacked it and Issels' work there.

As early as 1952, an investigator was sent to the clinic. He was so impressed with what he found that he warned the doctor that he had been sent to find evidence against Issels in order that the clinic could be closed. He warned Issels of his powerful enemies. The investigator's favorable report to the German Ministry of Health was "mysteriously lost."

By 1958, the American Cancer Society had "blacklisted" Dr. Issels. The long arm of Mary Lasker's oppressive organization had reached into a number of countries by then, intimidating honest researchers. According to *Dr. Issels and his Revolutionary Cancer Treatment* by Gordon Thomas:

> "By 1958, scientists from a dozen countries had visited the clinic. . . . They asked that Issels make no public reference to such visits. They quite properly feared cancer societies in their own countries would terminate research grants if it became known they had actually called on a man blacklisted by the powerful American Cancer Society."

A year later, a professor from Holland did a statistical analysis of Issels' "full cures" and published a report in a German medical journal. There was an outcry from the German Cancer Society which soon began a whispering campaign that the cured cases were faked.

One year later, Dr. Issels was arrested on trumped-up charges. He was put into a special cell block which contained only convicted murderers. A judge admitted to Issels' lawyer that "If we can convict Issels of fraud, we have a list of over 100 doctors we can also arrest—and then the internal cancer therapy is finished."

It took four years and two trials before Dr. Issels was found innocent. The clinic had been closed. Thousands who might have been saved by his treatment died.

In 1968, the British Broadcasting Corporation (BBC) became interested in Dr. Issels and his reopened clinic. They invested a substantial sum of money in investigating him. Outside medical experts were hired. Former intelligence officers were hired. BBC accounting experts examined the clinic's books. They concluded that Issels was legitimate and his treatment of cancer "a considerable improvement on what is usually offered."

The fact that the BBC was considering a television program on Dr. Issels brought forth the full fury of the British, American and German cancer officials. (Censorship has always been their strongest weapon.) One leading American cancer authority who had agreed to travel to Germany in order to conduct an independent assessment for the BBC hastily withdrew "after talking to the American Cancer Society."

A highly regarded British cancer authority was so impressed with what he found that he attempted to do a double-blind study in England. The English authorities turned him down. Soon his own research grants were threatened. The American Cancer Society, the German Cancer Society and the International Union Against Cancer in Geneva exerted pressure. The reason: "Issels had appeared on the American Cancer Society blacklist."

When the BBC investigated and sought an explanation from the American Cancer Society, the ACS was "reluctant to explain in detail its blacklisting of Issels."

The television production, titled "Go and Climb a Mountain," was scheduled for airing on March 17, 1970. It was "mysteriously" cancelled.

Then, on October 18, 1970, eight months later, a British newspaper discovered what was happening. A front page article in *The Observer* headlined, "Cancer Film Banned by BBC." Slightly more than two weeks later, on November 3, 1970, because of the enormous public pressure which followed, the BBC aired "Go and Climb a Mountain."

An audience of 14 million watched. But the orthodox cancer authorities weren't about to admit they were wrong. They sent a five man team to Germany to investigate. Two of those sent were adamant opponents of Issels. Only two of the members spoke German and they weren't cancer specialists. The report was another lie. It claimed the cures were imaginary. Misdiagnosed. Years of work and thousands of cases all misdiagnosed. The editor of *New Scientist,* a respected journal, ridiculed orthodox medicine for its "vicious intolerance of an unorthodox outsider . . ."

The story of Dr. Issels is especially instructive because it reveals how orthodox medicine operates and how far it will go to silence or stop an opponent. Lies were common in the Issels case. Falsified evidence was used to imprison Issels. The judicial system was perverted to incarcerate Issels with convicted murderers. Pressure was put on cancer experts not to conduct objective investigations. Television executives were coerced. That a conspiracy existed was admitted by a judge.

It is important to recognize also that Dr. Issels was a particularly tough, dedicated doctor. Individual American doctors under similar pressure who encountered the ACS or the AMA or attorney generals directed by medical officials usually would not be able to withstand such force. They would surrender. If not they lost their medical licenses. They went to jail. They left the country.

In the story of Issels is a blueprint of how the tyrannical elements of the Medical Mafia operate. There are more "smoking guns" in this tale than most. It is important to keep this in mind when considering other alternative therapies which have been suppressed. It is important to remember Issels when defenders of the orthodox treatments claim that NCI or FDA found documents supporting alternative therapies to be "inadequate." Cover-up has been the name of the game in cancer therapy for a long, long time.

It is also important to know that Dr. Issels' approach to terminal cancer treatment can be expanded and combined with new (and old) approaches. Issels' book describing his method is titled *Cancer: A Second Opinion.* Judith Glassman's *The Cancer Survivors* and Gordon Thomas' *Dr. Issels and His Revolutionary Cancer Treatment* are also valuable. Issels has provided a wonderful model which other doctors with terminal cancer patients can follow. If they have the guts.

Gary Null's 1988 book *Complete Guide to Healing Your Body* includes the following critical point regarding Dr. Issels:

"While skeptics may mutter about 'spontaneous remissions,' it remains true that three independent studies of Dr. Issels' medical research conducted by highly reputed experts have confirmed a 16.6 percent cure rate among all the terminal patients treated . . . a figure that no doctor or hospital anywhere in the world comes close to matching . . .

"To understand the significance of this figure, it is necessary to recall that all these patients were terminal, already given up on by conventional medicine. In the United States, for example, such a patient has virtually *no* chance of survival, let alone of cure."

# Appendix E
# Experiment #54—The Apricot Kernel Soup Cover-up

The National Cancer Institute (NCI) paid an independent research institute to conduct a very expensive study of laetrile in 1973. It was a poorly controlled experiment that apparently produced the results which NCI wanted. NCI could have determined early the optimum dose of laetrile for numerous experimental mice and concentrated its attention on the optimum dose. For some mysterious reason, it chose not to do so despite having a huge budget for the study.

What the NCI-sponsored statisticians and distortion-experts did to achieve the desired test result was mix together in the statistical results *all* those mice which got (1) poisonous doses of laetrile, (2) low doses of laetrile, and (3) the optimum dose of laetrile.

When the mice which got the optimum dose were compared with the control group which got a sugar injection (placebo), the results were astonishing. According to a fellow of the Royal Statistical Society in London, there was "one chance in four billion that the results occurred by chance."

The key to the cover-up can be found in *experiment #54*. Thirty male mice all at a point where their tumors were about to kill them got three days of injections of laetrile while a control group in the same condition got a placebo. Both groups got their shots on days 12, 13 and 14.

The first mouse to die in the control group died on day 12. The first mouse to die in the laetrile group died on day 21, nine days later!

The optimum date of dying—when the mice in either group died at their highest frequency—was similarly convincing. For the control group, it was day 18, with most mice dead on the same day. For the laetrile group, it was day 27, again a nine day spread!

The statistical expert who studied the results exclaimed:

"The NCI conclusions were a total distortion of science. The underdosed and the overdosed mice were combined with those mice receiving the optimum dosage. The trial was absolutely, absurdly dishonest. The U.S. taxpayers have a right to demand their money back. NCI is an absolutely corrupt, inept, incompetent organization distorting the truth in order to support their own image and own budget."

The research institute which conducted the expensive mice test which "disproved" laetrile was the Southern Research Institute of Birmingham, Alabama.

The outstanding model for future, honest laetrile studies was provided by Dr. Harold Manner, Chairman of the Biology Department at Loyola University in Chicago. He published over 60 peer-reviewed scientific papers and authored six college level science textbooks. From 1979 to 1988, the Manner Clinic in Mexico treated 4,000 patients and documented the progress of each patient.

The Manner Clinic used laetrile in conjunction with a complete therapeutic program because Dr. Manner traveled to clinics in a number of countries and found laetrile was effective only when used in conjunction with a complete program involving detoxification, enzymes, vitamins, DMSO, etc.

Dr. Manner died in 1988. His book, *The Death of Cancer,* is recommended.[151]

# Appendix F
# **Germanium**

Germanium was discovered by a German chemist, Clemens Winkler, in 1886. An organic derivative was synthesized in 1967 by scientists associated with Kazuhike Asai, Ph.D. of Japan. Asai's compound, known as Ge-132, was fervently promoted by him as a miracle treatment for cancer and as a general health enhancer. As Asai wrote in his 1980 book *Miracle Cure: Organic Germanium* (Kodansha/Harper & Row):

> "A 54 year old company employee was diagnosed as having cancer of the lungs . . . doctors prescribed a 500 mg daily dosage of the germanium compound. An X-ray photograph taken five weeks later showed absolutely no trace of cancer. . . . Numerous cases of recovery from various other cancers are on record . . . Aside from the fact that the germanium compound stops the activity of cancer cells and halts the growth of tumors, its most promising characteristic is the capability of halting metastasis, or the spread of cancer cells . . .
>
> "Germanium proved to be particularly effective in treating leukemia among children and while in many cases the disease could be arrested, just as many children entirely recovered."

Laboratory experiments with Ge-132 at the Robert Koch Institute in Berlin showed Asai's compound to be "highly effective" in making cancer cells revert to normal (Sandra Goodman, *Germanium: The Health & Life Enhancer*). A German company eventually developed its own, different version: Sanumgerman. However, as interest grew, so did trouble.

A number of companies began marketing "organic germanium." Fantastic health claims were accompanied by the assurance that Ge-132 was "completely non-toxic." Carefully synthesized Ge-132 apparently was safe. But without strict quality controls, the public couldn't be sure what it was buying. Kidney failure was reported from Japan as a result of germanium dioxide contamination in germanium preparations.

Germany banned germanium sales to the public. A scandal emerged from the marketing of questionable germanium formulas and high profits in England. The Germanium Institute of North America disbanded. Dr. Asai died, with some of his most controversial scientific claims having been disproved by objective researchers.

And yet critical questions remained. Why, given the terrible increase in lung cancer (31% increase in America from 1973 to 1987) did not qualified cancer researchers carry out *clinical* research in America with high quality Ge-132? Why, given the "anecdotal" but remarkable lung cancer and leukemia cures documented in Japan, did not the National Cancer Institute *immediately* commission some "quick" trials? Why? Why? Why? Because the people in charge were incompetent, and cared only for "business as usual" and their own pet projects, rather than providing therapies that work, even though the science was poorly understood.

Parris M. Kidd, Ph.D., who co-founded the Germanium Institute of North America, sadly summarized the germanium tragedy in the November 1990 *Townsend Letter for Doctors*.[48] Among his observations, the following are most pertinent:

> "Excellent Ge-132 preparations are available commercially, but the manufacture of pure Ge-132 demands significant investment of expertise, time, and money . . .
>
> "The future of this product has been seriously endangered by over-blown health claims, and by dangerous QA (quality assurance) practices that allowed toxic compounds of germanium to reach consumers . . .
>
> "Pure Ge-132, taken in small quantities (less than 2,000 mg/day) appears unlikely to pose any danger to the health of the consumer. Impure Ge-132, taken in whatever quantity, poses a clear risk that could be life-threatening, as occurred in Japan. The overall toxicity of the germanium element is low, but Ge can be highly toxic if built into the wrong molecular confirmation . . .
>
> "Whatever the path chosen toward making Ge-132 'legal' for human health applications, it is sure to require sizeable expenditures. The attractive aspect of the *pure* Ge-132 product is its diverse range of benefits and its excellent benefit-to-risk ratio."

# Appendix G
# **The Exploiters**

It is unfortunate that a number of people have used the publication of *The Cancer Cure That Worked* and the first edition of *The Healing of Cancer* to exploit the public. These exploiters have used the growing interest in Royal Rife's cancer curing technologies to make quick profits by claiming their black boxes were "Rife instruments" or were advanced models incorporating Rife's discoveries with those of other energy medicine pioneers. As a result of this duplicity, many desperate cancer patients have spent thousands of dollars on bogus "Rife instruments" or what was passed off as an improvement. By including a copy of either or both of my books or simply "riding on the interest in Rife," these multilevel marketers and fly-by-night operators left the impression with desperate and sometimes near-destitute people that their cancers could be effortlessly and painlessly cured. Many of these sales people are equivalent to unethical used car salesmen or boiler room telephone con men (and women). Equally guilty are the engineers, doctors and companies which endorsed the black boxes or produced them while "making no claims," yet using the name Rife in their advertising literature. The exploiters knew full well that an unsophisticated person with cancer who read either book would eagerly plunk down $600 or $1500 or as much as $6000 for a chance at something which would cure the illness.

Sadly, in most cases, the cancer patients lost precious time—3 or 4 months—before recognizing that they had been swindled in a clever marketing scheme. People died because they had faithfully used the worthless black boxes instead of orthodox or alternative, non-conventional cancer therapies which actually worked. But the black box makers and promoters ignored the damage they had done, banking the profits or

191

sometimes proclaiming that the money was going to "research."

One cancer patient used an expensive black box for a couple of months, then decided to have a Cat Scan to see what the effects were. The Cat Scan showed his cancer was metastasizing. When he and his family complained to the exploiters, they were told not to worry because the cancer was "breaking up." He died and the company refused even to refund the patient's money.

Another person with a benign tumor was given assurances by the maker of a black box that his instrument could eliminate it. The person innocently accepted. The benign tumor became malignant after "treatment" with the engineer's so-called super device.

Another exploiter admitted that if people didn't follow his program exactly, then the instruments he marketed could *cause* cancer. Nevertheless, he bragged about the thousands of instruments he intended to dump on the market.

Still another exploiter purchased an over-the-counter frequency generator for $200, attached a plate with the name "Rife" to the generator and then, presto!, proceeded to sell the generator for $2000. Even though the foreign manufacturer warned, "Do not use for human beings, dangerous," the man continued to sell them. His written justification? He had the right to make a profit and "had nothing to lose." But his clients sure did.

Law enforcement officials are investigating a number of these exploiters. Hopefully the worst offenders will be jailed for the serious crimes they have committed against their neighbors.

Anyone who has been exploited or knows someone who has been injured, died or simply been financially "ripped off" is encouraged to provide me with the facts. See the address at the end of this Appendix.

Anyone who has had *documented* success with a black box in reversing their cancer or eliminating a tumor is also encouraged to contact me in order that their good fortune can be shared with others. Please provide copies of medical records. Statements or claims without supporting evidence are of no value. Your records with your names will be kept confidential and will not be circulated unless you provide special permission.

Anyone contemplating the purchase of a black box that is being promoted as a "Rife Frequency Generator" or "Rife Resonator" or a "third or fourth generation" improved super duper whiz pro whatchamacallit should insist on documentation from at least 5 cancer patients cured by the so-called wonder device. And at least telephone access to the fortunate ex-cancer patients. Don't believe that such folks don't exist who will "stand up" *if* the black box did what the exploiters claim. Once the potential purchaser of a black box has checked and actually talked with real people who have documented records of a cure, then the potential purchaser must compare the kind of cancer, the prior treatment and other critical variables.

It is a tragedy that the resurrection of Rife's work did not bring about the careful laboratory and clinical reconstruction by qualified scientists and physicians which was the original aim. Instead, four or five people who could have served all of humankind chose to interfere in order to promote their own questionable devices, using the Rife name and making outrageous claims which time has proved to be either lies or terrible miscalculations.

Remember, if the real Rife's science ever becomes available again, the majority of people with cancer who use Rife's technology will be cured in 3 months or less. At the present time the phony devices just don't get those results.

Therefore, I urge my readers to be particularly skeptical of so-called "Rife" or "Rife-like" or "better-than-Rife" black boxes, no matter who promotes them, especially those who claim they have the "secrets." Let solid, documented results be the standard, not multi-level marketing falsehoods, misrepresentations and barefaced lies.

Barry Lynes

---

Readers who have a genuine need to contact Barry Lynes may do so at the address below. Please enclose a self-addressed, stamped, business size envelope.

Readers who have any information regarding a cancer patient or anyone else who was deceived into purchasing a "Rife" instrument should know that Barry Lynes welcomes any help that would contribute to putting these exploiters out of business.

Anyone who is (1) genuinely motivated and (2) possessing real assets or noteworthy talents which can contribute to a non-profit (foundation) or commercial development of Rife's or other non-conventional cancer therapies should feel free to contact Barry Lynes at the address below. However, this invitation does not extend to private practice physicians or chiropractors simply looking for an instrument to use in their "business." It also does not apply to "engineers" who believe they'd like to investigate this new world. I've wasted too much time with all three "professions."

Barry Lynes
P.O. Box 4186
Laguna Beach, CA
92652

# Notes

1. Peter Barry Chowka, "The National Cancer Institute and the Fifty Year Cover Up," *East-West Journal*, January 1978.
2. Ben Fitzgerald, *Congressional Record*, August 28, 1953.
3. David Rorvik, "A Defense of Unorthodoxy," *Harper's*, June 1976.
4. Ruth Mulvey Harmer, *American Medical Avarice*, 1975.
5. Ruth Rosenbaum, "Cancer Inc.," *New Times Magazine:* 11/25/77.
6. Mark J. Green, *The Other Government*, 1975.
7. Ralph Hovnanian, *Medical Dark Ages*, 2128 Prospect Ave, Evanston, Illinois 60201. Suggested donation by author is $10. ($2 for postage would be helpful.) (It's worth at least $15-$20.)
8. Edward J. Sylvester, *Target: Cancer*, 1986.
9. Hardin Jones, "A Report on Cancer," 1969. Available at U Cal Berkeley library.
10. Michael Culbert, *Save Your Life*, Dunning Pub., Virginia Beach, VA.
11. Lawrence Surtees, "Getting Nowhere," *Globe and Mail*, Toronto, June 11, 1988.
12. Gary Null, "Medical Genocide Part 16," *Penthouse*, 1987.
13. Dick Richards, *The Topic of Cancer: When the Killing Has to Stop*, Pergamon Press, Oxford, England and New York, 1982.
14. John Cairns, "The Treatment of Diseases and the War Against Cancer," *Scientific American*, November 1985.
15. Robert K. Oye and M. R. Shapiro, "Reporting Results for Chemotherapy Trials," *Journal of the American Medical Association*, 262:2722, 1984.
16. J. D. Bailar and E. M. Smith, "Progress Against Cancer?" *New England Journal of Medicine*, May 27, 1986.
17. Dr. Herbert Ley, San Francisco Chronicle, January 2, 1970. Senator Edward Long, U.S. Senate hearings 1965. Both quotations are from Hovnanian's *Medical Dark Ages* (footnote #7).
18. Daniel S. Greenberg, "Report of the President's Biomedical Panel and the Old Days at the FDA," *New England Journal of Medicine*, May 27, 1976.
19. Len Guttridge, "How the U.S. Government is Blocking a Cancer Cure," *Saga*, May 1968. Also appeared in *March of Truth on Cancer*, The Arlin J. Brown Information Center, PO Box 251, Ft Belvoir, VA 22060

20. "The Strange Saga of a Pain Killer," *TV Guide*, July 26, 1980. Reprinted in Hovnanian (see footnote #7).
21. G. E. Griffin, *World Without Cancer*, page 451. Reprinted in Hovnanian (see footnote #7).
22. Pat McGrady Sr., *The Persecuted Drug: The Story of DMSO*, New York, 1973.
23. Lester A. Sobel, *Medical Science and the Law*, New York, 1977.
24. Peter Temin, *Taking Your Medicine: Drug Regulation in the United States*, 1980.
25. Raymond Keith Brown, *Cancer, Aids and the Medical Establishment*, New York, 1986.
26. *Cancer Scandal*, a one-hour videotape featuring Robert G. Houston, Patrick M. McGrady, Jr., and Ralph W. Moss. Available from: Patient Rights Legal Action Fund, 202 West 78th Street, #3E, New York, N.Y. 10024. Price: $29.95 plus $3 shipping (total $32.95). Make checks payable to IFCO-Patient Rights.
27. Theodore Haecker, *Journal in the Night* .
28. Paul Starr, *The Social Transformation of American Medicine*, New York, 1982.
29. Howard H. Beard, *A New Approach to the Conquest of Cancer*. Reprinted in Hovnanian (see footnote #7).
30. Wayne Martin, *We Can Do Without Heart Attack,*1983. Reprinted in Hovnanian (see footnote #7).
31. M. Layne, *The Koch Remedy for Cancer*. Reprinted in Hovnanian (see footnote #7).
32. Ken Ausubel, "The Troubling Case of Harry Hoxsey." *New Age* magazine, July-August 1988. Also see Judith Glassman, *The Cancer Survivors*, New York, 1983 and Harry Hoxsey, *You Don't Have to Die*, New York, 1956.
33. Realidad Products, PO Box 1644, Santa Fe., N.M. 87504, Tel: 505-983-8956.
34. Gary Null, "Medical Genocide Part 8," *Penthouse*.
35. Norman Fritz, *Healing, Journal of the Gerson Institute*. Reprinted in Hovnanian (see footnote #7).
36. Rex Dalton, "Physician liked the challenge," *The San Diego Union*, March 9, 1987.
37. Peter Barry Chowka, "The Cancer Charity Rip-Off," *East-West Journal*, July 1978.
38. Walter S. Ross, *Crusade: The Official History of the American Cancer Society*, New York, 1987.
39. James T. Patterson, *Dread Disease*, 1987.
40. Samuel Epstein, *The Politics of Cancer*, 1978.
41. Lucy Eisenberg, "The Politics of Cancer," *Harper's*, November 1971.
42. Maryann Napol, *Health Facts*, The Overlook Press, Lewis Hollow Road, Woodstock, New York, 12498, 1982.
43. Ralph Moss, *The Cancer Syndrome*, New York, 1980.

44. Daniel S. Greenberg, "X-Ray Mammography—Background to a Decision," *New England Journal of Medicine*, September 23, 1976.
45. Maurice S. Fox, "On the Diagnosis and Treatment of Breast Cancer," *JAMA*, Feb 2, 1979.
46. Petr Skrabanek, "False Premises and False Promises of Breast Cancer Screening," *The Lancet*, Aug 10, 1985.
47. Edward Shorter, *The Health Century*.
48. Robert G. Houston, *Repression and Reform in the Evaluation of Alternative Cancer Therapies*, New York, 1987. Robert G. Houston, 115 East 86th St., New York, N.Y. 10028. Reprinted in *The Townsend Letter for Doctors*, 911 Tyler St., Port Townsend, WA 98368.
49. Gary Null, *Complete Guide to Healing Your Body Naturally*, McGraw-Hill, 1988.
50. Patrick McGrady Jr., *Newsday*, September 30, 1984. Reprinted in Hovnanian (see footnote #7).
51. *March of Truth on Cancer*, The Arlin J. Brown Information Center, PO Box 251, Ft Belvoir, VA 22060.
52. Scott Lucas, *The FDA*, Celestial Arts, Millbrae, CA, 1978.
53. Bob Owen, *Roger's Recovery from AIDS*, Davar Publications, PO Box 6310, Malibu, CA 90265 ($14.95 plus postage).
54. Judith Glassman, *The Cancer Survivors*, New York, 1983.
55. Kiichiro Hasumi, *Cancer Has Been Conquered*, Maruzen Co., Ltd., Tokyo 1980. Available from Price-Pottenger Nutrition Foundation, 5871 El Cojon Blvd, San Diego, CA 92115, Tel: 619-582-4168.
56. Robert A. Netterberg and Robert T. Taylor, *The Cancer Conspiracy*, 1981.
57. W. M. Crofton, *The True Nature of Viruses*, 1936.
58. George Melcher, testimony before Congressman Molnari's committee, January 1986.
59. Gary Null and Leonard Steinman, "The Vendetta Against Dr. Burton," *Penthouse*, 1986.
60. Robert O. Becker, interview in *Complementary Medicine*, March/April 1987.
61. Floyd Weston, interview in *Public Scrutiny*, February 1981.
62. George Lakhovsky, "Curing Cancer With Ultra Radio Frequencies," *Radio News*, February 1925.
63. William Laurence, "Crile Advances Life Ray Theory as Medical Basis," *New York Times*, October 9, 1933.
64. Newell Jones, "Dread Disease Germs Destroyed by Rays: Claim of San Diego Scientisit, Cancer Blow Seen After 18-Year Toil by Rife," *San Diego Evening Tribune*, May 6, 1938 (Repeated in *San Diego Union*, May 7, 1938.) (Additional article *Evening Tribune*, May 11, 1938.)
65. "$250,000 Fire Razes Mystery Workshop," *New York Times*, March 13, 1939, page 34.
66. Arthur Yale, "Cancer," *Pacific Coast Journal of Homeopathy*, July 1940.

67. Barry Lynes, *The Cancer Cure That Worked: 50 Years of Suppression,* Marcus Books, Box 327, Queensville, Ontario LOG 1R0, Canada, 1987 ($10.95 includes postage).

68. Robert O. Becker and Andrew Marino, *Electromagnetism and Life,* State University of New York Press, 1982.

69. Albert Szent-Gyorgyi, *Electronic Biology and Cancer,* Marcel Dekker, New York and Basel, 1976.

70. Julian N. Kenyon, *21st Century Medicine,* Thorsons Publishers, England, 1986.

71. Franz Morell, "MORA-Therapy: The Patient's Own Electromagnetic Oscillations as a Principle of Therapy," lecture.

72. S. Sullivan, D. Eggleston, J. Martinoff and R. Kroening, "Evoked Electrical Conductivity on the Lung Acupuncture Points in Healthy Individuals and Confirmed Lung Cancer Patients," *American Journal of Acupuncture,* Vol 13, No. 3, July-September 1985.

73. Wolfgang Ludwig, "Biophysical Diagnosis and Therapy in the Ultrafine Energy Range," Reports No. 1 and 3.

74. Veronica Strang, "Homeopathy: A Fitting Remedy," *The Missing Link,* March/April 1986, Toronto.

75. Malcolm Browne, "Unlikely Results of Experiment Published in Scientific Journal," *The New York Times,* June 30, 1988.

76. Stephen Strauss, "New Discovery May Explain Basis for Homeopathy," *The Globe and Mail,* Toronto, June 30, 1988.

77. Dana Ullman, "Recent Homeopathic Research Startles Scientists," *Townsend Letter for Doctors,* Aug/Sep 1988. For address, see footnore 48.

78. John Langone, "The Water That Lost Its Memory," *Time,* Aug 8, 1988.

79. C. S. Muir and D. M. Parking, "The World Cancer Burden: Prevent or Perish," *British Medical Journal,* Vol 290, 5 January 1985.

80. Annals of New York Academy of Sciences, October 11, 1974.

81. Thomas E. Jones, "Communicating with One's Self: A Wave of the Future," Fourth General Assembly of the World Future Society.

82. Gordon Thomas, *Dr. Issels and His Revolutionary Cancer Treatment,* Peter H. Wyden Publishers, New York, 1973.

83. Eustace Mullins, *Murder by Injection: The Story of the Medical Conspiracy Against America,* 1988. Available from PO Box 1105, Staunton, VA 24401 ($15.00).

84. Jan Stjernsward, "Decreased Survival Related to Irradiation Postoperatively in Early Operable Breast Cancer," *The Lancet,* November 30, 1974.

85. *New England Journal of Medicine,* 8 January 1981.

86. Daniel Greenberg, "A Critical Look at Cancer Coverage," *Columbia Journalism Review,* January-February 1975.

87. *A Complaint Against Medical Tyranny,* Committee for Freedom of Choice in Medicine, 146 Main St., Suite 408, Los Altos, CA 94022.

88. *The Cancer War,* Pub Broadcasting System. Reprinted in Hovnanian (see footnote #7).

89. J. W. Gofman and E. O'Connor, *X-rays: Health Effects of Common Exams*, San Francisco, 1985.

90. Charles B. Inlander, Lowell S. Levin and Ed Weiner, *Medicine on Trial*, 1988.

91. Joel Griffiths and Richard Ballantine, *Silent Slaughter*, Chicago, 1972.

92. Ernest Sternglass, "Observations in the Light of Chernobyl," speech delivered in New Haven, Connecticut, May 30, 1987.

93. Michael Gold. *A Conspiracy of Cells*, New York, 1986.

94. Robert C. Atkins, *Dr. Atkins' Health Revolution*, 1988, Houghton Mifflin Co., Two Park St., Boston, MA. 02108., $18.95.

95. Jon Rappoport, *AIDS Inc.*, Human Energy Press, 370 W. San Bruno Ave, Suite D, San Bruno, CA 94066.

96. Steve Connor, AIDS: Science Stands on Trial: One Year in Pursuit of the Wrong Virus," *New Scientist*, 12 February 1987.

97. Robert C. Gallo and Luc Montagnier, "AIDS in 1988," *Scientific American*, October 1988.

98. *Omni*, December 1988.

99. Charles Linebarger, "Tragedy at San Francisco General," *San Francisco Magazine*, July-August 1988.

100. R. Yarchoan, H. Mitsuya and S. Broder, "AIDS Therapies," *Scientific American*, October 1988.

101. Bruce Nussbaum, *Good Intentions: How Big Business and the Medical Establishment Are Corrupting the Fight Against AIDS*, 1990.

102. Alan Cantwell, *AIDS: The Mystery and the Solution*, 1983, Aries Rising Press, PO Box 29532, Los Angeles, CA 90029.

103. Stephen S. Hall, "Gadfly in the Ointment," *Hippocrates*, Sep/Oct 1988.

104. Taped interview available from Summit University, Dept V-200, Box A, Livingston, MT 59047-1390; Tel: 406-222-8300.

105. Gus G. Sermos, *Doctors of Deceit and the AIDS Epidemic: A View from the Inside*, GGS Publishing, 202 Jackson St, McComb, MS 39648.

106. John Mattingly, *Microscopy, Bacteriology and Gaston Naesson's Biological Theory*, January 1986.

107. Monica Bryant, "Microbiology at a Turning Point," *Journal of Alternative Medicine*, March 1986.

108. Peter Farb, *Living Earth*, New York, 1959.

109. *Business Week*, September 16, 1986.

110. Royal R. Rife, *History of the Development of a Successful Treatment for Cancer and Other Virus, Bacteria and Fungi*, San Diego, 1953.

111. Daniel Koshland, "The Mind of a Microbe," *Science Digest*, October 1983.

112. *Brain-Mind Bulletin*, Nov 1987, PO Box 42211, 4717 North Figueroa St., Los Angeles, CA 90042.

113. Robert O. Becker, *The Body Electric*, 1985.

114. Brendan O'Regan, "Healing, Remission and Miracle Cures," *Institute*

*of Noetic Sciences*, May 1987, 475 Gate Five Road, Suite 300, P.O. Box 97, Sausalito, CA. 94966-0097.

115. O. C. Gruner, *Study of Blood in Cancer*, Montreal, 1942.

116. Al Schaefer, *Health's Enemy is a Microbe Including Cancer*, International Association of Cancer Victims and Friends, Apollo Chapter, 40 Privateer Road, N. Palm Beach, FL 33408. Gregory's book is titled *Pathogenesis of Cancer*, 1948, 1952, 1955.

117. Florence Seibert et al, "Bacteria in Tumors," New York Academy of Sciences, Series II, Vol. 34, No. 6, pages 504-533, June 1972.

118. Florence Seibert, personal communication, 1987.

119. John Mattingly, *Commentary on the Followers of Antoine Bechamp*, 1988.

120. Jane Brody & Arthur Holleb, *You Can Fight Cancer and Win*. Reprinted in Hovnanian (see footnote #7).

121. Bruce Halstead, "The Halstead Cancer Battle," *Health Consciousness*, June 1986.

122 Lillian Newberry, "The Controversy Over Unproved AIDS Drugs," *Toronto Sunday Star*, March 27, 1986.

123. Katie Leishman, "AIDS and Syphilis," *The Atlantic*, January 1988.

124. Alan R. Gaby, "Institutionalized Ignorance," *The Townsend Letter for Doctors*. (See footnote #48 for address.)

125. Michael Culbert, *Vitamin B-17: The Fight for Laetrile*, 1974.

126. See *Business Week*, Sep 22, 1986, *The Toronto Globe and Mail*, May 28, 1988 and *The Wall Street Journal*, May 1988.

127. Lawrence Surtees, "Firm Denounced Over Cancer Therapy," *The Globe and Mail*, Toronto, May 28, 1988.

128. Paul Feyerabend, *Science in a Free Society*.

129. William D. Kelley, *One Answer to Cancer*. This book is out of print, but much of the same material can be found in Fred Rohe, *Metabolic Ecology: A Way to Win the Cancer War*, 1982. Available from Wedgestone Press, PO Box 175, Winthrop, KS 67156. Also see Tom and Carole Valentine, *Medicine's Missing Link*, Thorson's Publishers, 1 Park St., Rochester VT, 05767, USA.

130. Ben Bagdikian, *The Media Monopoly*.

131. G. Edward Griffin, "The Hoax of the Proven Cancer Cure," *Cancer Control Journal*, Vol 5-6, 1977/1979. Reprinted in Hovnanian (see footnote #7).

132. Herbert Bailey, *A Matter of Life or Death: The Incredible Story of Krebiozen*. Reprinted in Hovnanian (see footnote #7).

133. G. Edward Griffin, *World Without Cancer*. Reprinted in Hovnanian (see footnote #7).

134. Emerson Hartman, *Cancer News Journal*, 1977. Reprinted in Hovnanian (see footnote #7).

135. William C. Heuper. Reprinted in Hovnanian (see footnote #7).

136. Glen Kittler, *Laetrile: Nutritional Control for Cancer with Vitamin B-17*. Reprinted in Hovnanian (see footnote #7).

137. J. Richard Crout, quoted in *Spotlight*, January 18, 1982. Reprinted in Hovnanian (see footnote #7).

138. Harold Ladas, "The War on Cancer," *Holistic Medicine*, Vol 3, London, 1988.

139. Richard Ericson, *Cancer Treatment: Why So Many Failures?*, GE-PS Cancer Memorial, Publisher, Park Ridge, IL, 1979.

140. E. W. McDonagh, "Alternative Medicine Holds Answers Establishment Seeks," *The Spotlight*, July 9, 1990.

141. "MRMC Report, May 1990," Medical Research Modernization Committee, P.O. Box 6036, Grand Central Station, New York, N.Y. 10163-6018, Telephone: 212-876-1368.

142. The International Association of Cancer Victors and Friends, Inc., 7740 W. Manchester, Suite 110, Playa del Rey, CA 90293. Active chapters exist in California, Florida, Georgia, Illinois, New York, Texas, Washington state, Canada and Australia.

143. Christopher Bird, *The Life and Trials of Gaston Naessens*, 1990. Available from Marcus Books, P.O. Box 327, Queensville, Ontario, L0G 1R0, Canada, Tel: 416-478-2201.

144. Ralph Moss, *The Cancer Industry*, Praeger House, 1989, Nuremberg quote from World Medical Association, Ethics and Regulations of Clinical Research, R.J. Levine: Urban & Schwarzenberg, 1981.

145. Susan B. Anthony University Journal, October 1975, cited in Hovnanian (footnote #7).

146. Bruce Halstead, *Amygdalin Therapy*, 1972.

147. Dorothea Lynch & Richard Evans, *Exploding Into Life*, Aperture Books, 20 East 23 St, New York, N.Y. 10010 in association with *Many Voices Press*.

148. Irwin Bross, *Crimes of Official Science: A Casebook*, Biomedical Metatechnology Press, Buffalo, N.Y., 1988.

149. Stephen Kaufman and Betsy Todd, *Perspective on Animal Research*, Vol 1, 1989, ($8.00 paperback and $15.00 hardcover). See footnote #141 for address.

150. Evelleen Richards, "The Politics of Therapeutic Evaluation," *Social Studies of Science*, SAGE, London, Newbury Park and New Delhi, Vol 18, (1988), 653-701.

151. Harold Manner, *The Death of Cancer*, Metabolic Research Foundation, P.O. Box 4280, San Ysidro, CA 92072.

# Index

## A

# F

# G

Lakhovsky, George 70-71
Lasker, Albert 39, 40, 53
Lasker, Mary 39, 40, 41, 42, 48, 53, 115, 116, 153, 182
Lee, Royal 120-121
Ley, Herbert 17
Livingston-Wheeler, Virginia 125, 153
Ludwig, W. 79

## M

Mammograms 9, 44-47, 168-169
Mandel, E.E. 1
Marino, Andrew 76
Mattingly, John 119, 126
Mayo Clinic 146
McGrady, Pat Jr. 51, 52, 132, 137, 145, 158
McGrady, Pat Sr. 21, 50-51, 125
McKenna, Joan 106-108
Media coverage 14-15, 25, 147-148, 153-155
Medical Dark Ages 163
Medical Freedom 140-142, 148, 149
Melcher, George 65
Memorial Sloan-Kettering 1, 42-44, 48, 61, 62, 66, 92-96, 115,
   125, 143, 153, 173
Metzenbaum, Howard 64-65
Microbes 117, 119, 121, 122, 126
Microwave 178
Microzymas 118-120, 126-127
Montagnier, Luc 97-99, 102, 110
MORA 78-80
Morell, Franz 78-79, 81
Moss, Ralph 43, 44, 62, 143, 154
Mullins, Eustace 30, 94
Mycology (fungus) 119-120

## N

National Cancer Institute (NCI) Chapter 5, pages 55-68
   Newsday reports on conflict of interest 2
   Burton cover-up 2, 63-67
   Chemo & surgery recommendation 10, 14
   Protected fiefdom 25
   Hoxsey conspiracy 32, 174
   Tool of American Cancer Society 41, 44, 45

## U

Ullman, Dana  82
Unions (labor)  138
Unproven Methods List  49-51, 143, 183
Urine test  31, 166

## V

Virus  59-60, 72, 74, 77, 90, 119, 122
   AIDS virus  97-101, 108, 109, 110
Vitamin C  76, 146
Voll, Reinholdt  77-78

## W

Waldthaler, Urban  106
War on Cancer  41-44, 115, 119
Watson, James  1, 4
White, Theodore  157
Woodruff, Judy  14

## X

X-rays  See radiation

## Y

Yale, Arthur  74-76